# THE
# SOAPMAKER'S
# COMPANION

## A COMPREHENSIVE GUIDE WITH
## RECIPES, TECHNIQUES & KNOW-HOW

SUSAN MILLER CAVITCH

*A Storey Publishing Book*

STOREY

Storey Communications, Inc.
Schoolhouse Road
Pownal, Vermont 05261

*. . . Let us lay aside every weight, and the sin which doth so easily beset us, and let us run with patience the race that is set before us . . . .*

Paul the Apostle
New Testament, Hebrews 12:1

## DEDICATION

For Matt, who encouraged me six years ago when I felt called to this adventure
and who encouraged me again as I felt called to bow out.
And for Peter, Jenny, Adam, and Mary, who have kindly shared soap with me
and who make the choices easy ones.

*The mission of Storey Communications is to serve our customers by publishing practical information that encourages personal independence in harmony with the environment.*

Edited by Deborah Balmuth
Cover design by Meredith Maker
Cover and interior illustrations by Laura Tedeschi
Text design and production by Susan Bernier
    (Based on original design by Carol Jessop, Black
    Trout Design)
Indexed by Northwind Editorial Services

Storey Publishing books are available for special premium and promotional uses and for customized editions. For further information, please call the Custom Publishing Department at 1-800-793-9396.

Printed in the United States by R.R. Donnelley

10 9 8 7 6 5 4 3 2

**Library of Congress Cataloging-in-Publication Data**

Cavitch, Susan Miller, 1959–
    The soapmaker's companion : a comprehensive guide with recipes, techniques & know-how / by Susan Miller Cavitch.
        p.   cm.
    "A Storey Publishing Book"
    ISBN 0-88266-965-6 (pb : alk. paper)
    1. Soap.   I. Title
TP991.C395
668'.124—dc21                                         97-5139
                                                          CIP

# Contents

# ACKNOWLEDGMENTS

This book was my editor Deborah Balmuth's idea. She and I had tossed around the idea of an eventual second edition to *The Natural Soap Book,* but a more advanced soapmaking book felt right to Deborah before I knew for myself. Deborah, your sense of order leaves the book reader-friendly, and your gentle manner makes collaboration enjoyable. To the extent that an editor can enhance or diminish the author's experience, your sweet spirit made the process a pleasure. Thank you.

Dr. Matthew White is a kind chemist who was willing to be interrupted to help a relative stranger in the middle of a busy day. As comfortable discussing covered bridges as esters, he is a patient teacher. Thank you, Matt, for helping me stay on track. If mastery involves stewardship, your generous sharing of the gift leaves you a fine steward.

Terrianne Taylor is a fourth-generation soapmaker. Both of her great-grandmothers were soapmakers. Her maternal grandmother, Paula Ohnesorge, lived on a small dairy farm in northern Minnesota where she saved her fat drippings all year long for the annual soapmaking and leached her own lye from wood ashes. Like so many of her generation, she worked hard, recycled everything, and wasted nothing.

When Terrianne was a child, her grandmother taught her how to make soap. Terrianne can still recall the smell of sparkling-clean laundry hanging on the line just after it had been cleaned with her grandmother's laundry soap. Of course, Mrs. Ohnesorge's laundry soap was also her bath soap and her shampoo. Her animal-based soap contained no fanciful nutrients, yet Terrianne remembers a mild bar of soap with a fresh smell. The soap was made in orange crates lined with seed sacks. Some batches were permeated with the scent of the pine needles spread between the crates and the sacks; the unscented batches had a clean, fresh scent of their own.

Eva Mae and Cliff Pelton, Terrianne's mother and father, continued the soapmaking tradition into adulthood. They made their own bath and laundry soap at home, and once a year, their German Lutheran country church group gathered to produce 500–600 pounds of soap for World Relief. Donations of various fats and oils poured in all year long, and then over a two-day period, everyone came together to make soap in 5-quart ice cream pails. (Yes, they made soap in plastic containers, and yes, they and Mrs. Ohnesorge made tallow soap at 75–95°F (24–35°C)!) The soap was sent to impoverished countries along with the quilts and blankets the group had sewed throughout the year.

Terrianne has been around soapmaking all of her life, but recently made it her family business. She and her husband, Jim, operate the Pretty Baby Herbal Soap Company in North Carolina. It had been years since she had made soap when Jim arrived home from work to find her stirring something out in the backyard on the glider. He knew then and there that he was in trouble. What he didn't know was that a little over a year later, Terrianne would have a successful soap business and he would leave his job to join her.

Both Jim and Terrianne say they have learned to run a business just as they learned to parent — by trial and error. Years of being around soap has left her with good instincts, so most of Terrianne's experiments work first time around. Though her mother, grandmother, and great-grandmothers all made soap, they did not use the selection of vegetable oils available to today's soapmaker. Terrianne was on her own as she designed an all-vegetable formula. But her mother and father continue to share the soap-making adventure with her, passing along wonderful tips and stories, and I have a hunch that she gets a little help from beyond, from those women who made soap for function and never imagined swirls of violet and bars by the name of Medicine Man.

Terrianne has developed lovely soaps with rich, creamy lathers and beautiful colors. Her marbled bars are the prettiest I've seen. She uses over a dozen ingredients in each batch. In place of plain water, she uses herbal infusions. Her refrigerator is filled with gallons of green and brown concoctions that are fortunately hard to mistake for lemonade or orange juice. With names such as Sassy Singapore, Sudzy Navel (Orange, That Is), My Sister's Soap (she has red hair), Kaleidosoap, and Oats & Goats, her soaps reflect the fun she and Jim are having together. Terrianne's interest in natural skin care has led to a line of complementary products: Scented Sun-Dried Sea Salts for the Bath, Mineral Herb Scrubs, Shampoo and Body Bars, and a new line of creams and lotions. Pretty Baby Herbal Soap offers a soapmaking kit packed in a reusable wooden tray, with a variety of refills available for making different kinds of soap (see "Suppliers" section of appendix for an address).

Thank you, Terrianne, for the fun names you gave my soap, for your generous nature, and for a story that inspires others to be matriarchs and patriarchs.

# PREFACE

I wrote my first book, *The Natural Soap Book,* in response to my feeling that there were too many people seeking guidance on this topic from involuntary mentors. Updated soapmaking formulas were not widely available, and instructions were varied and contradictory. My goal was to pass along all that I thought the reader needed to know to make good soap, within the confines of limited space. I tried to make my methods accessible, condensing information only to avoid becoming too technical or too long, or when it seemed that I might supply more detail than readers' interest could support. But I have found this latter fear to be unfounded. I will run out of knowledge before readers' interest wanes. Details are what soapmakers crave.

I expected people to enjoy soapmaking, since I enjoy it so much, but I have been overwhelmed by the high level of interest and experimentation. I knew that people wanted to know how. I hoped they would want to know why. But now people are asking, "Why not?" I should have seen this coming. After all, pioneer crafts foster a pioneer spirit. The appeal of the quiet, useful art draws us in, the satisfaction of self-reliance keeps us involved, and the spirit of wonder drives us forward. Figuring out how to make soap doesn't end the quest; it just better equips us to advance the craft.

All fields experience periods of resurgence, growth, and leveling off until the next phase of development. Soapmakers are still in the period of renewal, and creative people from all over are contributing to this particular wave. Soapmaking forums are growing online. Soapmaking businesses are cropping up everywhere. Some hobbyists make soap for themselves; others are trying to supplement or even supplant family incomes. Beginners soon become teachers, encouraging newcomers and enlarging the community of interest.

Some people want to know only what they need to know to accomplish a certain objective. Others want to know more even when it is not clear that the knowledge will ever be useful. *The Soapmaker's Companion* is written and organized (as described on pages 8 to 10) for both types of people.

# INTRODUCTION

Before jumping into new ideas, some old ones are worth reviewing. There are many different kinds of soap; this book and *The Natural Soap Book* focus on only one kind: all-vegetable, cold-process soap made as naturally as possible. The goal is to create a mild soap that cleans and moisturizes without synthetic intrusion.

Individuals are uniquely positioned to make better soap than companies that are mass-producing the product. Mass-producers must concern themselves with profit, which can be an inhibiting factor. Synthetic ingredients are accessible, stable, and economical, so they are often used in place of richer natural ones. When industrial manufacturers do incorporate organic nutrients, the percentages are often insignificant — eye-catching on the label and inconspicuous in the soap. A quick glance at the labels reveals the highly synthetic nature of most body-care products. Consumers have little or no understanding of the products' ingredients. Many people react negatively to one product or another and are left to find the culprit responsible for the rash, an irritation, or the dry skin. The home soap-maker can balance frugality and quality and often meet family skin-care needs better than industry can.

## BACK TO BASICS

Though *The Soapmaker's Companion* is best read as a sequel to *The Natural Soap Book* or any other primer, it includes enough of the basics to be read as a stand-alone work. The following quick overview summarizes the basic points more exhaustively explained in such a primer.

## What Is Soap?

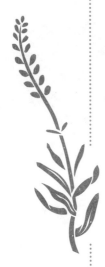

Soap is simply made, though the chemical reaction is complex. Chemically, an acid (the fats and oils) and a base (a solution of sodium hydroxide and water, also called lye) react to produce soap and glycerin. The process is called saponification, and as the fats and oils and the lye solution come into contact with one another and react, they are saponifying, or making soap. The mixture gradually changes from a separated mixture of heavier, watery lye and lighter fats and oils to a thicker, uniform mixture. The soap mixture is ready to be poured (for most recipes) when it has thickened to the point when a bit of soap drizzled from the spatula onto the surface of the soap leaves a trail (a pattern) for a moment before disappearing beneath the surface. This state of readiness is known as a "trace," since only a trace of the pattern remains when the soap is ready. An ingredient that is to be added "at the trace" is not incorporated into the soap pan until the trailings are recognized as such by the soapmaker.

A variety of acids and bases and a series of processes produce soap, but homemade bars are made using easily accessible materials and a simple process called the cold-process — once the sodium hydroxide solution is added to the melted fats and oils, no external heat is required to keep the soapmaking reaction going. The heat of the ingredients is plenty to drive the reaction to completion. "Cold" does not mean cold; it was coined as a relative term, comparing it to the more common hot soapmaking temperatures produced when heat is applied.

The two most critical chemical components of the soapmaking process are contact and heat. The acid and the base must first come together before they can react; heat encourages movement and fluidity, and stirring ensures it. Soap is ready to pour once the ingredients have been evenly dispersed in a thick, stable emulsion. Further reaction can take place later provided that the acid and the base are positioned closely enough to connect and react.

## How Does Soap Clean?

Soap helps clean in two ways: it helps water "wet" the surface to be cleaned, permitting water to reach more of the surface; and it connects the dirt to the water, permitting the dirt to rinse away.

A soap molecule consists of a chain of carbon, hydrogen, and oxygen atoms — arranged with a distinct head and tail. The head is attracted to water and the tail is attracted to dirt and oil. Soap cleans because these opposing parts connect dirt to water, permitting it to be rinsed away.

Soap also helps water to wet better. Water beads up on fabric and skin because its molecules are tightly bonded and resist being broken apart. The molecules cling to one another in droplets and do not soak the surface. This is where soap intervenes as a surface-active agent — something that breaks apart these droplets and helps them wet the skin or fabric. When soap molecules are combined with water, their hydrophobic tails (the hydrocarbon chains) squeeze together in a small space, in an effort to get as far away as possible from the water and as close as possible to one another. The heads of the soap molecules (the carboxyl portion) are attracted to the water and form a spherical wall around their fleeing tails. The soap forms a film on the surface of the water that holds the heads and tails in position. The action of these heads and tails on the water's surface breaks the surface tension, forces the water into the fabric or skin, and allows the soap's lather to develop.

Once the soap molecule has helped water do its job, it next removes dirt and grease. The oil-loving tail of the soap molecule is attracted to oil and grease. It first embeds its tail into the dirt. As the water-loving head of the soap molecule pulls toward the water, the dirt is dislodged as it remains attached to the tail of the molecule. The tail of the soap molecule then holds the dirt in suspension, away from the skin or fabric, until a rinse washes the dirt and the soap away.

## SOAPMAKING INGREDIENTS

The workhorse ingredients in soapmaking are the fats and oils, sodium hydroxide, and water — the acid, the base, and the solvent to dissolve and disperse the base.

Before the fats and oils are blended with the lye solution, they must be in liquid form. Normally, this involves melting any solid fats before mixing them with any of the liquid oils. (See Chapter 4 for a more in-depth discussion of the most common fats and oils used by the soapmaker.)

Though water does play a role in the chemistry of soapmaking, its more visible role is as a solvent; dry sodium hydroxide sprinkled over a mixture of fats and oils would not come into contact with enough of the oil to make soap, but when it is dissolved in water, the water carries it to all corners of the pan to meet all of the fat and oil molecules. Remember that it is the uniting of the fats and oils with the sodium hydroxide that produces soap.

Sodium hydroxide is often referred to as lye. Lye has two meanings. It is the solid form of a caustic alkali, and it is also the water solution in which a caustic alkali has been dissolved. Soapmakers can use the terms lye and sodium hydroxide interchangeably, but to avoid confusion, I distinguish between the two as follows. I most often call the chemical sodium hydroxide, "sodium hydroxide," and the sodium hydroxide/water solution, "lye."

Sodium hydroxide in its present form was not around throughout most of soap's history. The caustic alkalis (bases) used for soapmaking were potash leached from wood ashes, and various carbonates produced from the ashes of seaweeds and land plants. The soaps were harsh and soft, and often rather unpleasant. Not until the 1700s was a way discovered to make caustic soda (sodium hydroxide) economically.

Sodium hydroxide (NaOH) comes in a variety of forms, but the solid flake and bead are most practical for the home soapmaker. Local or mail-order chemical companies are the best sources for larger quantities of sodium hydroxide; bulk purchases are most economical, but be mindful of safe storage and seal tightly to avoid rock-hard clumps of material. In the presence of moisture in the air, the sodium hydroxide flakes absorb the water and clump into solid chunks. For small quantity purchases, many supermarkets carry Red Devil lye in plastic containers often shelved next to the Drano in the aisle with cleaning products. *Be careful not to use Drano as a lye substitute.* Also, squeeze the can of lye to be sure that the product has not been exposed to moisture. A crunchy can should be left behind.

Until recently, soapmakers did not stray much from the standard soapmaking ingredients: tallow, palm oil, coconut oil, soy oil, palm oil, sodium hydroxide, and water. Milk, honey, and oatmeal added the special touches. Today the possibilities are limited only by purity and stability, and the list of options cannot be confined to the page. The two pages that follow list a variety of soapmaking fats, oils, nutrients, scents, exfoliants, colorants, and preservatives, some of which were discussed in *The Natural Soap Book* and some that are included in *The Soapmaker's Companion.* The list is provided to inspire new combinations.

Combining these ingredients to make good soap should not be a random process. There is a logic and the logic can be learned. Any of the vegetable oils listed as nutrients can also be included from the start of the soapmaking process as majority soapmaking oils. Often, the high cost of these oils limits them to superfatting oils added at trace. Less stable nutrients like aloe vera gel and honey are added at trace to retain more of their active, healing properties. Exfoliants like oatmeal, cornmeal, and poppy seeds are added at trace to the thicker soap for an even and permanent suspension of material. Scent is always added at trace, because these oils, which are very different from fatty oils, cause the soap to begin setting up (congealing and hardening). The natural preservatives listed are optional and are added to the melted fats and oils before they are blended with the lye solution.

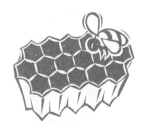

## Pure Essential Oils

The highly concentrated volatile oils obtained from plants, which carry the scent and the beneficial properties of the particular plants. They are volatile because they evaporate quickly at room temperature when exposed to air.

## Fragrance Oils

Synthetic imitations of pure essential oils. Fragrance oils do not offer the botanical properties found within pure essential oils and they can cause soap to set up prematurely, but some contribute lovely scents to soap.

# SOAPMAKING INGREDIENTS

| FATS AND OILS | NUTRIENTS |
| --- | --- |
| almond (sweet) oil | almond (sweet) oil |
| avocado oil | aloe vera |
| calendula oil | apricot kernel oil |
| canola (rapeseed) | beeswax |
| cocoa butter | borage oil |
| coconut oil | calendula oil |
| cottonseed oil | carrot oil |
| hazelnut oil | castor oil |
| hemp seed oil | cocoa butter |
| hybridized oils | copaiba balsam |
| jojoba oil | egg |
| kukui nut oil | evening primrose oil |
| lard | hazelnut oil |
| olive oil | hemp seed oil |
| palm kernel oil | honey |
| palm oil | lanolin |
| peanut oil | lecithin |
| safflower oil | macadamia nut oil |
| sesame oil | milk |
| soybean oil | neem oil |
|   (vegetable | pine tar |
|   shortening) | propolis |
| sunflower seed oil | pumpkin seed oil |
| tall oil | rose hip seed oil |
| tallow | rosin |
| wheat germ oil | sesame oil |
| | shea butter |
| | tea tree oil |
| | wheat germ oil |

### SCENTS

| | |
| --- | --- |
| anise | myrrh |
| basil | neroli |
| benzoin | nutmeg |
| bergamot | orange |
| caraway seed | patchouli |
| cassia | Peru balsam |
| cedarwood | petitgrain |
| chamomile | pine |
| cinnamon | rose |
| clary sage | rosemary |
| cloves | rosewood |
| coriander | sandalwood |
| dill | tangerine |
| fennel | thyme |
| frankincense | Tolu balsam |
| geranium | tonka bean |
| grapefruit | vanilla |
| juniper berry | vetiver |
| lavender | ylang-ylang |
| lemon | |
| lemongrass | |
| lime | |
| litsea cubeba | |
| marjoram | |
| mint | |

## COLORANTS

alkanet root
annatto seed
beetroot
   powder
beta-carotene
black-eyed
   Susan
brazilwood
calendula
   blossom
caramel
chlorophyll
cinnamon
cochineal
cocoa
comfrey
cutch
elderberry
ginseng
goldenrod
goldenseal
henna
licorice root
madder root
mimosa
paprika
resins
rose hips

safflower
saffron
Saint-John's-
   wort
seaweed
soapwort
sumac berry
turmeric
ultramarines
walnut
wheat germ
yarrow

## EXFOLIANTS

alfalfa meal
almond meal
cornmeal
flaxseed meal
jojoba meal
juniper berry meal
millet seeds
oatmeal
poppy seeds
seaweed
tapioca pearls

## PRESERVATIVES

carrot root oil
grapefruit seed
   extract
tocopherols

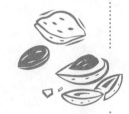

## ABOUT THIS BOOK

*The Soapmaker's Companion* has been written for the reader who is looking for much more than a "how-to" book. Only my limitations and the unknown keep me from sharing more. My goal was not only to pass along formulas, warnings, and tips, but also to share a body of academic knowledge with the more curious. Those readers who have already made soap can probably set up the work area and begin making the soap in Chapter 1, though I recommend reading Part I first for pointers. Beginners and those soapmakers who do not make soap regularly benefit from a careful review of the basics. The best soapmaking usually results from a wide range of knowledge; the best soapmaker is more often the one who understands the unique properties of different fats and oils, the best way to incorporate a color, and the more subtle changes to look for during the soapmaking process. Soap can be made without understanding the realm of possibilities, but the soapmaker is more limited.

Beginning soapmakers should start with the recipe for Soap Essentials Bar II. This formula is simple and the soap is simply wonderful. Making a basic soap familiarizes the new soapmaker with the process — the order of steps and the look of the soap as it progresses from one stage to the next. (Colors and additives can camouflage the more subtle changes.) After a couple of successful batches of Soap Essentials Bar II, the soapmaker is ready to experiment with additions like cocoa butter, oatmeal, and colors. Once comfortable with substitutions and last-minute additions, the soapmaker can move to techniques such as layering and marbling. Transparent soap is, in my opinion, for the seasoned soapmaker who feels ready for a wildly different challenge. Once the basics are understood and recognized in the soap pan, experimentation is just a batch away. This play is the reward for disciplined study, and it is fun, safe, and wholeheartedly recommended.

Part I, "Soapmaking in the Kitchen," is divided into three subparts, Recipes, Ingredients, and Practical Know-How, and is filled with practical advice about how to make better soap. Part I is best reviewed in its

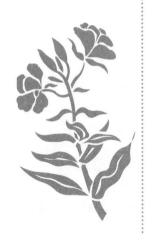

entirety before making soap. The recipes section describes the soap-making process, step-by-step; the ingredients section explains how oils, colorants, and scents can be innovatively used; and the practical know-how section helps you anticipate problems before they occur.

"Recipes" begins with Chapter 1, which features 29 recipes, ranging from a White Chocolate Mousse bar to a very special face and body cream to a few versions of laundry soap. Chapter 2 describes how to make visually impressive soaps. Chapter 3 teaches how to make transparent soap.

"Ingredients" starts with Chapter 4, which reviews the many common and uncommon soapmaking fats and oils and their charateristics. Chapter 5 identifies the available natural colorants and explains how to use them. Chapter 6 introduces some fragrance ideas from around the world.

In the subpart, "Practical Know-How," Chapter 7 explains how different soapmaking temperatures affect the process, the saponifying mixture, and the final bars. Chapter 8 identifies obvious and subtle signs of trouble and suggests remedies. Chapter 9 answers more than forty of the most common questions.

Part II, "Soapmaking in the Library," offers an intensive education about some of the science underlying soapmaking. You could skip Part II and still make wonderful soap, but don't. Chapter 10 discusses resins, what they are and how they might be used by the soapmaker to add beneficial properties or darken color. Chapter 11 describes minerals and clays, what they are, what they might add to the soap, and whether they are safe to use. Chapter 12 explains what is meant by a saturated fat or oil versus an unsaturated oil and how the soapmaking process and final soap bars are affected by the degree of saturation. Chapter 13 explains the chemistry, not just what you need to know to calculate with SAP values, but a discussion of what is really happening at the atomic level.

Part III, "Soapmaking in the Marketplace," is written for those soapmakers who want to share soapmaking with others — either online or by starting a soap business. Chapter 14 introduces you to the various soapmaking forums on the Internet where you can share your knowledge and learn from others. Chapter 15 addresses some of the corporate and tax issues you need to consider when starting a business. Chapter 16 examines your insurance options. And Chapter 17 surveys the federal regulation of soapmaking and warns you of the stringent regulations involved if you are classified as a cosmetics producer rather than a soapmaker.

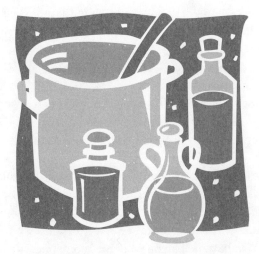

# Soapmaking
# in the Kitchen

PART 1

# CHAPTER 1
## Recipes for Vegetable-Based Soaps

My greatest pleasure in soapmaking is designing new recipes, unveiling the experimental batches, and seeing that they worked. In a world of assembly-line burgers — a world that rewards the economic efficiency of mass production and honors sameness — I embrace the opportunity to invent colors, mold shapes, change textures, choose skin-care attributes, and add fragrances.

Once you understand the basics you, too, can design your own signature bars. The reader who understands the chemistry of soapmaking has no need for someone else's recipes. Once you understand how to substitute one fat or oil for another, and what percentages to use of sodium hydroxide, water, various nutrients, and essential oils, reworking soap formulas is quick, easy, and fun. Do not feel limited by the recipes I offer — you can simply rework them to meet your preferences. You may like soaps made with cocoa butter or have a friend who loves oatmeal and honey goat milk soap. Maybe you know someone with allergies who over-reacts to scents and needs a soap without them.

Enjoy my recipes and have fun designing your own. Most likely, your favorite creations will be those that have been carefully and lovingly designed for your family and friends. Don't be surprised if before long your neighbors and friends are sharing personal skin histories with you. It's satisfying to respond with a soap or a cream that offers some relief.

## SPECIAL FEATURES OF THESE RECIPES

Each of the following recipes produces fifteen 4-ounce (113-gram) bars of soap. Feel free to double or triple a recipe as desired. You may have to adjust the amounts of water slightly when using significantly higher soapmaking temperatures, due to the evaporation that occurs at high processing temperatures (see chapter 9, page 177). The ratios of the other soapmaking ingredients do not change if batches are increased or decreased.

## To Superfat or Not to Superfat

I continue to experiment with my formulas in an attempt to learn more about the effect of any one adjustment on the final bar. My preference is for a hard bar that is mild, moisturizing, and cleansing, with a rich, generous lather. My goal has always been to find ways to increase any one of these traits without significantly lessening any one of the others. I walk a fine line at times.

One of the most important factors involves the maximum percentage of sodium hydroxide permissible in a mild bar of soap. For years I took a 15.5 percent discount from the amount of sodium hydroxide required for complete saponification. Since then I have continued to test the possibilities and the limits, and I have worked my way to a 10 percent discount. I apply slightly lower discounts to those recipes that incorporate a meaningful percentage of hemp seed oil, the most unstable oil I've worked with to date, and to those that incorporate ground nut meal, aloe vera gel, or whole grains.

## The Soapmaking Temperature

The recipes in this book can tolerate a wide range of temperatures, though I have suggested my favorite range for most recipes — between 80°F and 100°F. Recipes that require a more limited range specify the temperatures under the heading, "Temperatures."

## The Stir

All of the recipes in this book are perfectly suited to a freestanding electric mixer, though those who love a quiet workout can make any of the following recipes by hand. Just be sure to stir as quickly and forcefully as the *lower* speeds of a mechanical mixer.

**Superfat**

To superfat a soap is to leave unsaponified oils in the final bars for the mildest soap. Unsaponified oils do not form compounds with the other soapmaking components but, instead, remain in their original form in the bar as emollient ingredients.

**Discount**

A reduction, expressed as a percentage, from the amount of sodium hydroxide required for a complete saponification. When a discount is applied, a percentage of fats and oils are left unsaponified in the final bars as moisturizing ingredients.

## Tracing

The state at which soap has thickened sufficiently to scent and then pour into molds. Most batches have traced sufficiently at a light trace, when a portion of the soap drizzled from the spatula leaves a trace of the pattern before sinking back into the mass. For layered soap, I recommend a full trace — allowing the soap to thicken *just* to the point when the trailings of soap begin to remain on the surface. Learn to recognize the first signs of trace to avoid the overly thick soap caused by delay that makes it difficult, if not impossible, to scent and pour level bars.

### THE IMPORTANCE OF ADEQUATE STIRRING

*Note:* The most common stirring mistakes relate to stirring the soap inadequately. When soap is poured too soon before the trace, or when it is stirred too slowly or inconsistently, lye can be found in the final bars as solid pieces, liquid pockets, or powdery residue. Though all of the following formulas can easily be stirred by hand, the mechanical stir more reliably incorporates all of the lye.

One important thing to remember: Stirring affects tracing time. Until I decreased the size of my batches, I had never made soap using an electric mixer. Most of my 15-pound (6.8-kg) batches of soap take fifteen to twenty minutes to trace when hand-stirring. Because I enjoy the quiet process of making soap by hand, and the tracing time is short, I have never bothered using a mixer for these batches. However, when I cut the batch size to 5 pounds (2.3 kg) for the recipes in this book, and found myself testing many small batches in a day, I decided to experiment with a freestanding mixer. The consistent results I obtained reminded me how important it is to stir quickly. Since I hand-stir briskly and firmly, the mixer does not shorten my tracing times significantly. But for people whose hand-stirring is irregular, a mixer ensures a quick and consistent stir. It is especially useful in recipes that replace all of the water with milk; these soap mixtures must be stirred quickly and constantly for a smooth soap with a fine grain.

When hand-stirring, stir as quickly and firmly as possible, from the beginning to the end of the soapmaking process. Use a soapmaking pan large enough to accommodate occasional splashing. At first, when the soap mixture is more watery, your stir will be somewhat inhibited, though you can still stir quickly and firmly. Once the mixture begins to thicken, you can stir more and more quickly and forcefully. Five minutes or so into the soapmaking process, you can practically beat the soap back and forth and around and around. When hand-stirring less than 3 pounds (1.4 kg) of soap at a time, a wire whisk is helpful to ensure a quick, thorough stir.

If you are using a mixer, begin with a low speed (1). Then increase to setting 2 once the mixture thickens somewhat. Be sure to use a splash-guard. Closer to the end, you can go a little faster, but never use the high speeds — you might whip air bubbles into the soap mixture that will remain in your final bars. I rarely increase the speed above 2. (For more discussion of stirring, see chapter 9, pages 171–173.)

# EQUIPMENT

Ideal equipment for making 5-pound (2.3-kg) batches of soap:

***For mechanical mixing only:*** freestanding electric mixer, mixing
   bowl, paddle, and splash-guard
***For hand-stirring only:*** 8-quart (7.6-liter) enamel or stainless steel
   pot (the "soapmaking pan") and wire whisk
***For mechanical mixing or hand-stirring:***
- ◆ 3-quart (2.8-liter) stainless steel or enamel saucepan
- ◆ 2–3 quart (1.9–2.8 liter) heat-resistant glass bowl or pitcher
- ◆ 2 heavy-duty rubber or silicone spatulas
- ◆ Good-quality scale (preferably two scales — one measured in grams,
   one in ounces)
- ◆ One good-quality thermometer (0–220°F [18–104°C]; the quick-read
   type is best)
- ◆ Trays or molds (5 pounds, or 2.3 kg, of soap poured into a rectangular wooden tray that measures 15" x 6.85" [38 cm x 17.4 cm] produces
   fifteen bars of soap that measure 2.9" x 2.28"), or 7.6 cm x 5.8 cm —
   adjust as desired)
- ◆ Heavy-duty waxed freezer paper for lining the trays
- ◆ Masking tape to flatten the paper against the sides of the trays
- ◆ A sharp, thin paring knife for cutting and trimming the soap
- ◆ Safety goggles and gloves

## SAFETY EQUIPMENT AND CONCERNS

Everyone making soap should wear goggles
and gloves for protection. Purchase gloves
that are somewhat close fitting, allowing
you a degree of feel. Look for latex,
neoprene/latex, heavy plastic, or natural rubber gloves. Make sure that the

**A NOTE ABOUT MEASURING**
Do not measure ingredients by
volume (except for essential oils,
which can be measured by either
volume or weight). Weight is far
more reliable. A couple of soapmaking manuals offer formulas calculated by volume, but unless you're
feeling confident with this system,
it's worth recalculating the formula (carefully) into weight.

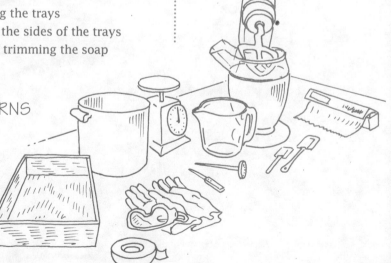

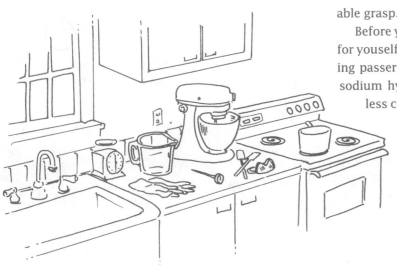

material isn't slippery; it's important to have a reliable grasp.

Before you begin, think about the safety concerns for youself, your family, your pets, and any unknowing passersby, keeping in mind the dangers of dry sodium hydroxide, the lye solution, and even the less concentrated soap within the pot. Pots and bowls should not be placed close to the edge of a counter or a table. Educate your family; put up warning signs; make sure that you'll be able to monitor the process from start to finish or wait for another time; and factor in all of the contingencies you can think of before deciding to proceed.

## EQUIPMENT MATERIALS TO AVOID

Soap may be fairly harmless and mild, but its components go through some very active, caustic stages before they are tamed. Equipment for the soapmaking process must hold up to these components at their nastiest. Lye eats through some materials instantly, and others over time. Cold-process soaps lose their caustic properties only after weeks of curing, so the equipment you use, from beginning to end, must weather varying concentrations of lye. Here are my recommendations for materials to avoid:

◆ Do not use anything made of aluminum, tin, iron, or Teflon, which are all corroded by lye.

◆ Avoid cast iron; seasoned iron pots deteriorate somewhat, discoloring the soap.

◆ Plastic becomes too weak and flexible in the presence of high temperatures (although heavy-duty plastic is better).

◆ Avoid wood. After using wooden spatulas for a couple of years, I switched to heavy-duty rubber or silicone ones, since the wood becomes soft, splintered (leaving tiny splinters in the soap pan), and impossible to thoroughly clean when constantly exposed to the caustic soda. Rubber or silicone spatulas are more expensive but last longer.

## Working with Sodium Hydroxide

Sodium hydroxide is highly reactive in its dry form or within solution. One bead of lye can burn right through layers of skin in the presence of just a hint of sweat. A splash of solution can burn or blind you and even eat into a butcher-block table.

This compound is worthy of our greatest respect and even greater caution. Sodium hydroxide is corrosive to all tissues. Accidentally swallowed, it causes serious internal injury and can be fatal. Even the weaker solutions can cause extensive damage.

Ingesting lye can be fatal if you do not act immediately. Past literature instructed people to neutralize any ingested sodium hydroxide with acids, such as lemon or lime juice, or vinegar, and then to drink a demulcent, such as egg whites or olive oil, which often induces vomiting. Poison control centers now urge people *not* to use this procedure and not to induce vomiting. Check with your local poison control center for the most up-to-date procedures. Be prepared to act should someone ingest sodium hydroxide. As of this writing, the recommended action is to give water only — 4 ounces (118 ml) for children and 8 ounces (236.6 ml) for adults — and to head to the hospital emergency room. In the case of eye exposure, irrigate the eyes with large quantities of running water and seek medical attention. Flood skin burns with large quantities of running water until the soapy, slippery feel disappears; then treat as you would treat any other burn.

The disposal of toxic chemicals is a critical issue for many businesses. The soapmaker must be aware of safe disposal, but we have the advantage of creating usable waste. Soap scraps can be recycled, and yesterday's lye can be used at another time if it is kept in a safely sealed container. Measurement errors can be corrected by adding more sodium hydroxide or water, as needed.

As your lye cools down for a few hours or overnight, be mindful of exactly where you set down the bowl. Remember to consider children, cats, dogs, and the level of activity in the room. Carefully think through location — as well as all other soapmaking steps — before you begin. It's better to cover all the bases, even those remote contingencies.

### WARNING

**Never** dispose of sodium hydroxide, lye, or raw alkaline soap without first researching local landfill regulations. These materials are toxic and hazardous.

## STEP-BY-STEP SOAPMAKING INSTRUCTIONS

The following basic recipe for Soap Essentials Bar II includes all of the steps needed to make any of the other recipes in this book. Please read these instructions carefully and completely before you proceed with any of the recipes.

### SOAP ESSENTIALS BAR II
*Makes 15 4-ounce (113-g) bars*

The original Soap Essentials Bar recipe, which appears in *The Natural Soap Book,* makes forty 4-ounce (113-g) bars and cannot be made in a noncommercial freestanding mixer. Many users of that recipe have expressed interest in a smaller batch, so they could either use a mechanical mixer or just make fewer bars at a time for a greater variety of soap. I have therefore revised my original formula to accommodate these requests.

201 grams sodium hydroxide
1 pound 3 ounces (538.7 g) distilled water
1 pound 5 ounces (595.3 g) olive oil
1 pound (454 g) coconut oil
14 ounces (396.9 g) palm oil
12 grams grapefruit seed extract (an optional
    preservative)
7 teaspoons (35 ml) pure essential oil or
    fragrance oil, optional

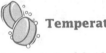

**Temperatures**

Fats and oils: 80–100°F (27–38°C)
Lye solution: 80–100°F (27–38°C)

Sodium Hydroxide Discount: 10%

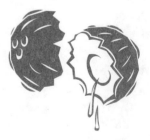

### Preparing the Work Area

**1.** Before beginning, set up your work area and required equipment.

**2.** Line a mold — a wooden tray or heavy cardboard box — with heavy-duty waxed freezer paper. Be sure to miter the corners and flatten the paper against the sides of the mold. Use masking tape to secure the paper to the mold without waves or wrinkles.

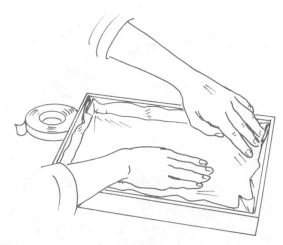

Lining the mold with waxed paper (step 2).

**3.** Measure out the essential oil, preservative, and extra nutrients, if desired, and set them aside in tightly sealed containers.

### Mixing the Key Ingredients

**4.** Put on your goggles and gloves. Weigh the sodium hydroxide and set it aside.

**5.** Set the glass container on the scale and add the distilled water; remove from the scale. Carefully add the sodium hydroxide to the water while stirring briskly with a rubber spatula. The fumes may overwhelm you after about ten seconds, so hold your breath while stirring as quickly as possible, then leave the room for fresh air. Return after two to three minutes to dissolve any remaining sodium hydroxide by stirring briskly. Do not wait longer or the beads will clump into a solid mass at the bottom of the bowl and resist dissolving.

The reaction will heat the lye solution to over 200°F (93°C), so set the bowl aside in a safe place to cool down to 80–100°F (27–38°C) (or your desired soapmaking temperature; see chapter 7). If you plan to cool the lye overnight, cover the container tightly to avoid weakening the solution.

**6.** While the lye is cooling, you can begin mixing the oils. Set the soapmaking pan (if hand-stirring) or the mixing bowl (if using a mixer) on the scale and add the desired weight of olive oil (or any other liquid oils, if you're using other soapmaking formulas). Then set the 3-quart (3-liter) saucepan on the scale and add the correct weights of coconut oil and palm oil (or any other solid fats or beeswax when you're using other soapmaking formulas).

Place the pan with the coconut and palm oils over medium heat until most of the solid pieces have melted (no stirring necessary). The few remaining chunks will melt from the heat of the pan. Pour the melted fats into the olive oil. Should you choose to use a natural preservative, add the grapefruit seed extract to the warm fats and oils, incorporating thoroughly. Let this cool to 80–100°F (or your desired soapmaking temperature; see chapter 7).

## Making the Soap

**7.** You are ready to make soap when the fats and oils and the lye solution have both cooled to the desired temperatures. If you have cooled the lye overnight and the temperature has dropped below this point, heat it up by setting the container in a sinkful of hot water. Oils can be heated over low heat on the stove for a short time, if necessary. Remove the pan from the stove once the oils reach 4°F (17.5°C) below your desired temperature; the heat in the pan will raise the temperature naturally.

**8.** Wearing goggles and gloves, slowly drizzle the lye into the oils, stirring as quickly as possible by hand. A freestanding mixer should be set at its lowest speed (setting 1) at this point in the soapmaking process. Continue to stir briskly, keeping as much of the mixture as possible in constant motion. When stirring by hand, stir briskly and forcefully throughout the entire soapmaking process, scraping the sides often to avoid a buildup of residue and to keep all of the ingredients in solution. A wire whisk works best for small batches. When using a mixer, keep the setting on the lowest speed until the mixture thickens; increase to setting 2 as it thickens even further.

When the lye is first added to the oils, the mixture is too thin and watery for an all-out beating, but stir as briskly as possible without splashing. About five minutes of continuous quick stirring produces a thicker, more uniform mixture that can gradually tolerate faster and stronger strokes. From this point until the soap is ready to be poured, the stir should be continuous, forceful, and brisk, and should reach all corners of the soapmaking pan.

Once a small amount of soap drizzled across the solution's surface leaves a faint pattern (called tracing) before sinking back into the mass, the soap is ready for the essential oils and nutrients, if desired. The soap should reach a trace within

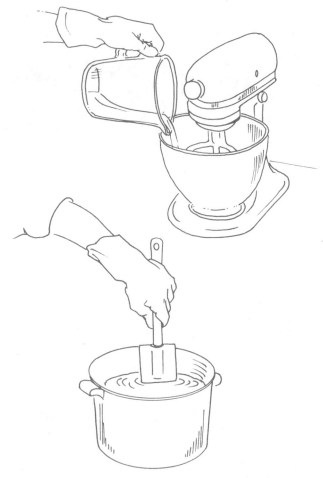

*Two stirring methods for combining lye and oils (step 8): In a mixer at low speed (top). Briskly by hand (bottom).*

ten to twenty-five minutes, when stirring by hand, and ten to fifteen minutes when using the electric mixer, if the stir is brisk enough (see box on page 23 regarding tracing time). Do not wait until the soap is thick enough for a pattern to remain on the surface (except when making layered soap) or the soap will harden too quickly once you add the essential oils; yet, be sure that all of the oils on the surface have been incorporated, leaving a uniform mixture.

**9.** Incorporate any desired nutrients, then immediately drizzle in the essential oils to scent the soap, stirring swiftly and thoroughly with a spatula. Stir for twenty to thirty more seconds, or for as little time as needed to fully incorporate the essential oils. Too much stirring causes streaking and seizing (a quick setup that makes it hard, if not impossible, to pour

the soap into the mold). Pure essential oils are usually cooperative; synthetic fragrance oils are more likely to streak and seize.

**Pouring into the Tray**

**10.** Once the oils are evenly distributed, quickly pour the soap into the mold. If you have periodically incorporated the soap from the sides of the pan for an even soap mixture, the entire pan — bottom and sides — can now be scraped clean with a spatula. If a residue has formed from an irregular scraping down of the sides of the pan, leave any crumbly pieces behind. The mixture should be smooth, with no lumps and a uniform texture and color. Watery or oily puddles signal a poorly mixed solution. Try to

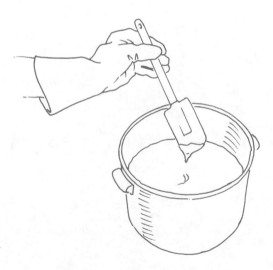

*Once the soap reaches a trace, add the essential oils and nutrients (step 9).*

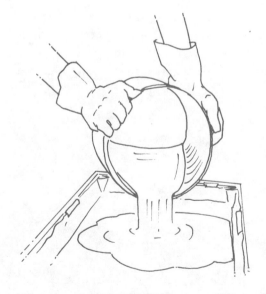

*Pour the soap mixture quickly into the mold (step 10).*

pour evenly from one end of the mold to the other for level, uniform bars.

If you see a change in texture, stop pouring. A last bit of soap mixture at the bottom of the pan that is watery and uneven indicates that your stirring process was not quite complete. Do not pollute the rest of your batch by adding this unsaponified portion. (See chapter 9, page 185.)

If your first attempt at pouring into the mold isn't quick enough and the mixture begins to set unevenly, use a spatula to spread it out to the corners. Keep in mind that the soap bars can be trimmed smooth once they are ready to be cut. When you follow this recipe carefully, you are unlikely to encounter this problem.

**Curing and Cutting the Bars**

**11.** Cover the filled mold with another frame, a piece of plywood, or a piece of heavy cardboard; cover with a blanket or two. Leave undisturbed for eighteen to twenty-four hours. Highly unsaturated soap formulas are best left for twenty-four hours; highly saturated soap formulas harden quickly (especially those with beeswax or cocoa butter) and can be opened sooner for easier cutting. The curing period is important, as the insulation allows the soap to heat up and saponify further.

**12.** Uncover the mold and set it away from drafts and cold temperatures for one to seven days, or until the soap is firm enough to cut. Don't wait until it's rock hard. (I actually cut the bars produced using this formula immediately after the insulation period.)

**13.** Using a ruler and a paring knife, lightly mark the slab into bars, being careful not to cut through. Once the bar lines look straight and uniform, cut lengthwise and crosswise through to the bottom of the mold. Holding the sides of the waxed paper, lift the entire layer of soap out of the mold. Stand the

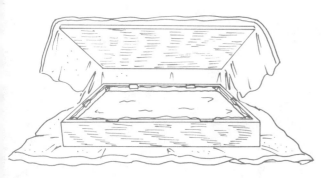

Covering and insulating the filled mold (step 11).

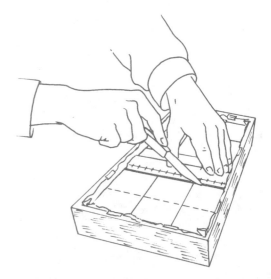

Cut the bars along the lightly marked lines (step 13).

block of soap on a table on one of its short ends and carefully peel the waxed paper downward toward the table, one row of soap at a time, removing the exposed bars before peeling down to the next row. Slice a ¹⁄₁₆-inch off the top of each bar to remove any powdery residue, if necessary (see chapter 9, pages 180–183.)

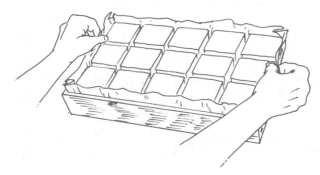

Lift the entire layer of cut bars out of the mold (step 13).

**14.** Lay the soaps, in a single layer, on plain brown paper grocery bags, or wicker or rattan place mats. Do not use bags imprinted with ink, as the bars are still alkaline and will pick up the dye. Set the soaps in a dry, well-ventilated room, protected from temperature extremes.

**15.** Allow the soaps to cure for three to four weeks, turning them over once to fully expose the other sides. This is an important period, because the soaps become dryer, harder, and milder. Wrap as you like, preferably in a breathable material. (For more discussion on curing, see chapter 9, pages 174–177.)

## A NOTE ON GRAPEFRUIT SEED EXTRACT

To produce the mildest soap, I do not completely saponify my soap mixture — that is, I use less sodium hydroxide than is required for a complete saponification, leaving what is called superfatted soap. Soap that isn't completely saponified is more vulnerable to spoilage, however. Grapefruit seed extract, a by-product of the citrus industry, is an all-vegetable antioxidant that extends the life of the superfatted bar by an additional six to twelve months. It contains vitamin C and glycerin and has proven to be antibacterial, antimicrobial, deodorizing, astringent, and antiseptic. I include this natural antioxidant in all of my formulas, but it is an optional ingredient. You can save yourself the cost of this expensive nutrient if you decide to take a smaller sodium hydroxide discount (see chapter 13, "The Chemistry of Soapmaking"), or if your soaps do not require lengthy protection.

**Note on tracing time:** Small batches made without grapefruit seed extract may take longer to trace. Always wait for a trace before pouring soap into trays to avoid streaks of solid lye inside final bars, or a thick, powdery layer on the surface.

## Temperatures

Fats and oils: 90–120°F (32–49°C)
Lye solution: 90–120°F (32–49°C)

Sodium Hydroxide Discount: 10%

---

### SUBSTITUTING OILS

You can substitute more accessible fats and oils for any that are difficult for you to purchase. Use the SAP values chart (see page 247) to adjust the sodium hydroxide.

You can also personalize your soaps by selecting a special color. Choose from the large selection of colors in chapter 5, "Using Natural Colorants," for those that fit the following recipes.

---

## EXPERIMENTAL BAR

This trial-sized batch makes one 5-ounce (141.75-g) bar of soap. The experimental bar is the key to avoiding waste and a tool that encourages far-out experimentation. When the only downside of a recipe is the loss of just a little time and a little expense, you are more likely to throw caution to the wind. Thanks to this baby batch, I've discovered that the less likely combinations can become favorites. When using tiny quantities of ingredients, metric measurements increase accuracy. The perfect mold is a recycled plastic cupcake or cookie liner.

16.8 grams sodium hydroxide
45.4 grams distilled water
42.2 grams olive oil
36.2 grams coconut oil
42.2 grams palm oil

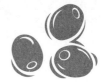

### Special Instructions

Tiny batches produce less of the initial soap that gets the soapmaking going, and they retain little heat; therefore, they take longer to trace. My 20-pound (9.1-kg) batches of soap take ten to twenty minutes to trace, and this little guy can take twenty to thirty minutes. I recommend using a freestanding mixer for the quickest, most consistent, most stress-free stir. Use a wire whisk when stirring by hand, to keep as much of the mixture as possible in constant, quick motion. You can use even higher temperatures than those listed above, but I have found that 140°F (60°C) temperatures do not provide faster results than 120°F (49°C) temperatures using this particular combination of fats and oils, and curdling is a risk. Add 1 gram grapefruit seed extract for a quicker trace.

**Note:** If testing a color, scent, or nutrient *quickly* is more important than the skin-care quality of the resulting bar, the Experimental Bar formula can be reworked to a more saturated formula that traces sooner and releases more quickly from the mold. Replace half or more of the olive oil with an equal amount of a combination of palm oil and coconut oil and adjust the amount of sodium hydroxide accordingly, using SAP values (see chapter 13).

## HEMPSTER'S DELIGHT

Hemp seed oil is new to the soapmaking scene. After years in relative obscurity, it has surfaced as a vegetable oil with some unique qualities (see chapter 4, page 101). Though a few soapmakers have been making hemp seed oil soaps for years, this oil is still somewhat of a mystery.

Hemp seed oil is one of the more effective skin-care oils, and it has a wonderful nutty smell that lingers. If it weren't so unstable, I would use it as 40 percent of the total fats and oils in a recipe. Unfortunately, only the strongest synthetic preservatives seem to protect large quantities of hemp seed oil, so I choose to incorporate a smaller percentage of it in my soap, take no more than a 10 percent sodium hydroxide discount, and double the dose of grapefruit seed extract.

A hemp seed oil soap wrapped in the loose weave of a hemp wash-cloth makes a nice gift.

203 grams sodium hydroxide
1 pound 3 ounces (538.7 g) distilled water
10 ounces (283.5 g) hemp seed oil
6 ounces (170 g) olive oil
1 pound (453.6 g) coconut oil
1 pound 3 ounces (538.7 g) palm oil
25 grams grapefruit seed extract (optional preservative)
7 teaspoons (35 ml) pure essential oil or fragrance oil, optional

**Temperatures**

Fats and oils: 80–90°F (27–32°C)
Lye solution: 80–90°F (27–32°C)

Sodium Hydroxide Discount: 10%

### A NOTE ON STUBBORN BATCHES

Use a stainless-steel whisk when hand-stirring the occasional stubborn batch. Whisk quickly and forcefully until the soap thickens.

# MRS. MINIVER'S MILK BATH

## Temperatures

Fats and oils: 80–100°F (27–38°C)
Lye solution: 80–110°F (27–43°C)

Sodium Hydroxide Discount: 10%

I've learned a little more about what I can and cannot control, so I no longer try to force hybrid tea roses to grow organically here in the hot, humid South. They cried for another home and I gave in. If a plant needs harsh pesticides and fungicides to stay alive, it probably doesn't belong where it is. Instead of fighting nature, I now grow old-fashioned roses and the shrub roses that tolerate the heat and humidity, and I make rose soap. Though their scents are more subtle, they represent to me the gifts that grow from humility and obedience.

Mrs. Miniver's soap will satisfy any winter craving when the rose garden is buried and dormant. Choose a good-quality rose oil for the truest scent. Ultramarine rose produces nearly the same mauve shade as the madder root in a milk soap. Without the milk, the ultramarine rose produces a less desirable shade of candy pink. I often make this soap without milk; the madder root colors it a beautiful red rose.

✓ 201 grams sodium hydroxide
12.8 ounces (362.9 g) distilled water
1½ tablespoons (22.5 ml) ground madder root
1 pound 5 ounces (595.4 g) olive oil
1 pound (453.6 g) coconut oil
14 ounces (397 g) palm oil
6.4 ounces (181.4 g) buttermilk
12 grams grapefruit seed extract (an optional preservative)
7 teaspoons (35 ml) rose oil

## SOAPMAKING NOTE

I prefer to make small batches of milk soap in a freestanding mixer for a more uniform blend. When hand-stirring, be sure that your stirring process is fast and force-ful and consistent to avoid a grainy soap mixture.

### Special Instructions

**1.** Dissolve the sodium hydroxide into the 12.8 ounces (362.9 g) of water. Immediately add the 1½ tablespoons (22.5 ml) ground madder root (ground finely in a coffee grinder). Just before adding the milk to the lye (see below), strain the solid madder root from the liquid lye. The pieces of root are too scratchy for inclusion in the soap.

**2.** When the lye solution and the melted fats and oils come close to the desired soapmaking temperature, gently heat the milk to the same temperature. Whisking quickly and firmly with a stainless-steel whisk, add the buttermilk to the lye solution. Once it is well blended, immediately begin pouring the lye/milk mixture into the melted fats and oils, beating briskly and firmly from start to finish.

## DIRT BUSTER

In general, I prefer smooth bars to grainier ones; I guess I'm not tough-skinned. Still, after a couple of early-morning hours of weeding, watering, pruning, and harvesting, gardener's soap does a better job of preparing me for public viewing. The exfoliants effectively remove dirt and sweat, while the soothing vegetable oils leave behind a moisturizing layer of protection on the skin. I like to scent this bar with herbal blends reminiscent of my time in the garden.

**Temperatures**

Fats and oils: 80–100°F (27–38°C)
Lye solution: 80–100°F (27–38°C)

Sodium Hydroxide Discount: 10%

191 grams sodium hydroxide
1 pound 3 ounces (538.7 g) distilled water
4 ounces (113.4 g) castor oil
8 ounces (226.8 g) wheat germ oil
5 ounces (141.75 g) jojoba oil
4 ounces (113.4 g) shea butter
1 pound (453.6 g) coconut oil
14 ounces (397 g) palm oil
12 grams grapefruit seed extract (an optional preservative)
7 teaspoons (35 ml) pure essential oil or fragrance oil, optional
¼ cup (50 ml) dried oatmeal (not instant), finely ground,
    or ¼ cup (50 ml) cornmeal

**Special Instructions**
At the trace, add the oatmeal or cornmeal and then the essential or fragrance oil.

## Temperatures

Fats and oils: 100°F (38°C)
Lye solution: 85°F (29°C)

Sodium Hydroxide Discount: 10%

## Exfoliant

Materials with irregular, somewhat scratchy textures used to release debris that collects on the skin's surface. As skin functions normally, sweat glands and sebaceous glands rid the body of waste and toxins. The skin also traps external pollutants on its surface in a barrier of sebum and sweat. Exfoliants, like oatmeal or cornmeal, add texture to soap lather, increasing the soap's cleansing qualities: the grainier lather releases dirt and dead surface skin while stimulating the healthier cells below. Always include moisturizing nutrients, like shea butter, cocoa butter, castor oil, or jojoba oil, in exfoliating formulas to avoid irritation and dryness. When using exfoliants, never rub with force. Soap and a little texture picks up debris without a heavy hand.

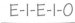

# E-I-E-I-O

Not surprisingly, farm life produces many soapmaking ingredients. The soapmaking farmer has access to some wonderful additions to the soap pot. Egg soap was one of the first soaps I made years ago, and it has been a favorite ever since. This is not only because our hens lay more eggs than we can pass along to neighbors, consume ourselves, or use as sharp weapons against slugs in the garden. Milk and eggs and lanolin also contribute richness and moisturizing qualities to any soap, and even just an ounce (28.35 g) of beeswax makes this a harder bar. I've left out the obvious — beef and mutton tallow and pork lard — but oatmeal is included as the hearty reward after all of those morning chores.

6.4 ounces (181.4 g) goat's milk
12.8 ounces (362.9 g) distilled water
218 grams sodium hydroxide
15 ounces (425.25 g) olive oil*
1 pound (453.6 g) coconut oil
8 ounces (226.8 g) vegetable shortening
15 ounces (425.25 g) palm oil
2 ounces (56.7 g) lanolin
1 ounce (28.35 g) beeswax
4 egg yolks, at room temperature
¼ cup (50 ml) dried oatmeal (not instant)
2 tablespoons (30 ml) ground bee propolis, optional
12 grams grapefruit seed extract (an optional preservative)
7 teaspoons (35 ml) pure essential oil or fragrance oil, optional

*Remove 1 cup (250 ml) of olive oil and set aside.*

**Special Instructions**

I recommend that this recipe be made in a freestanding mixer for a smoother grain, but this is optional.

In a coffee grinder, powder the oatmeal and the bee propolis into a fairly fine powder.

Add the sodium hydroxide to the water, whisking vigorously and continuously until the sodium hydroxide is completely dissolved. Allow to cool to 85°F (29°C).

Combine the beeswax with the coconut oil, vegetable shortening, palm oil, and lanolin, and heat until the beeswax is completely melted. Then add the olive oil (the original volume minus the removed portion) to the melted fats.

When the desired soapmaking temperatures are reached, warm the 1 cup of reserved olive oil to 85°F (29°C), then add the egg yolks, whisking forcefully to blend well. Heat the milk gently to 80°F (27°C). Drizzle the milk into the 85°F (29°C) lye solution, whisking briskly and constantly using a stainless steel whisk. Immediately add the lye/milk mixture to the 100°F (38°C) fats and oils, beating briskly.

After one to two minutes of blending, drizzle in the well-blended egg/olive oil mixture, stirring briskly the entire time to prevent the egg yolks from curdling. At the trace, add the oatmeal/propolis mixture.

**NOTE**

Egg yolk soap is best produced at lower soapmaking temperatures (80–90°F [27–32°C]) to avoid pieces of curdled egg in the final bars. To accommodate the high melting point/solidification point of the beeswax, the soapmaking temperatures for E-I-E-I-O bars are slightly higher.

## BABY GRAND

For years I have heard that less is more with respect to the skin care of babies and young children. Their skin often responds better to fresh air than to being coated with lotions and powders. The acid mantle of a baby's skin does not match an adult's and is easily irritated by adult skin-care products. I have found that babies need no more than the occasional bath using the mildest bar of soap. Unless a day has been particularly active (as baby days go), plain water is often just fine. To limit allergic exposures, avoid scent. You may miss it, but the baby won't. I promise.

194 grams sodium hydroxide
1 pound 3 ounces (538.7 g) distilled water
8 ounces (226.8 g) avocado oil
5 ounces (141.75 g) sweet almond oil
4 ounces (113.4 g) jojoba oil
4 ounces (113.4 g) shea butter

1 pound (453.6 g) coconut oil
14 ounces (397 g) palm oil
12 grams grapefruit seed extract (an optional preservative)
7 teaspoons (35 ml) pure essential oil or fragrance oil, optional

## BUILD ME A BUTTERCUP

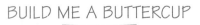

This is one of my favorite soaps. Annatto can be used to produce deeper shades of yellow and orange, but this recipe produces a warm, butter yellow. The yellow and orange safflower threads retain their color in the final bars for a bright contrast against the soft yellow background (see chapter 5, page 125).

1 pound 5 ounces (595.4 g) olive oil
1½ tablespoons (22.5 ml) annatto seeds or ⅛–¼ teaspoon annatto extract
201 grams sodium hydroxide
1 pound 3 ounces (538.7 g) distilled water
1 pound (453.6 g) coconut oil

14 ounces (397 g) palm oil
12 grams grapefruit seed extract (an optional preservative)
1½ tablespoons (22.5 ml) safflower threads
7 teaspoons (35 ml) pure essential oil or fragrance oil, optional

## Special Instructions

When using annatto seeds, remove ½ cup (125 ml) of the olive oil, add the seeds, and heat for thirty seconds on high in the microwave. Allow to steep to make annatto oil, stirring periodically to release the deep yellow color.

Just before adding the lye solution to the fats and oils, blend 5 tablespoons plus 2 teaspoons (10 ml) of strained annatto oil into the fats and oils mixture. Proceed as usual. When using the annatto extract, add it at the trace. Add the safflower threads just before you add the essential oil, at the trace.

# WHITE CHOCOLATE MOUSSE

This soap is another favorite. I've had more requests for this soap than for any other over the past year. I leave it white to accentuate the rich, creamy lather the added cocoa butter produces. Those individuals who are allergic to chocolate and cocoa butter should avoid this recipe, but others will love the silky yet greaseless feel of a soap made with a relatively high percentage of cocoa butter.

The smell of cocoa butter can overpower light herbal and floral scents, so I recommend scents such as almond, chocolate, vanilla, or Peru balsam (I use almond for white bars). Deodorized cocoa butter is available for those who want little or no scent.

**Temperatures**

Fats and oils: 100°F (38°C)
Lye solution: 100°F (38°C)

Sodium Hydroxide Discount: 10%

187.5 grams sodium hydroxide
1 pound 3 ounces (538.7 g)
   distilled water
11 ounces (311.85 g) olive oil
8 ounces (226.8 g) jojoba oil
1 pound (453.6 g) coconut oil

8 ounces (226.8 g) cocoa butter
8 ounces (226.8 g) palm oil
12 grams grapefruit seed extract
   (an optional preservative)
7 teaspoons (35 ml) pure essential
   oil or fragrance oil, optional

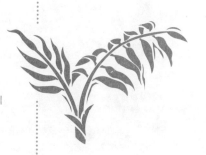

## Special Instructions

A meaningful percentage of cocoa butter produces a rock-hard soap. Cut this batch into bars immediately following the insulation period.

## SUNFLOWER SOAP

**Temperatures**

Fats and oils: 80–95°F (27–35°C)
Lye solution: 80–95°F (27–35°C)

Sodium Hydroxide Discount: 10%

When the more popular soapmaking oils, such as olive oil, are less plentiful and more costly, some soapmakers turn to hybridized oils (see chapter 4, page 116). Most unsaturated oils contain some saturated fatty acids that help the oil to saponify more readily, but high–oleic acid oils contain few to no saturates, so be prepared for longer tracing times. Soaps made with too high a percentage of high–oleic acid oils take longer to harden, but the following formula includes enough coconut oil and palm oil to keep the soap fairly well on track.

201 grams sodium hydroxide
1 pound 3 ounces (538.7 g) distilled water
1 pound 5 ounces (595.4 g) sunflower oil or high–oleic acid hybridized
    sunflower oil
1 pound (453.6 g) coconut oil
14 ounces (397 g) palm oil
12 grams grapefruit seed extract (an optional preservative)
7 teaspoons (35 ml) pure essential oil or fragrance oil, optional

**Special Instructions**
Consider adding yellow annatto oil (see chapter 5, page 125) and yellow and orange botanicals such as safflower and calendula for a stronger impact.

## SUSHI BAR

**Temperatures**

Fats and oils: 80–100°F (27–38°C)
Lye solution: 80–100°F (27–38°C)

Sodium Hydroxide Discount: 10%

I only had my friend Midori Abe here in Memphis with me for three years, but I didn't need long to know I'd made a lifetime friend. I have memories of time spent sharing cultures with one another, and I have the calligraphy her father sent to me. My children have her children as pen pals. I also have a lesson passed on from her grandmother to Midori to me: To not allow even one grain of rice to go to waste. I never wash sushi rice now without an awareness of the rice-free rinse water running down the drain. The Sushi Bar reminds me of Midori and her lesson of gratitude.

The idea for this soap came to me after a trip to the Asian market. The first time I made it, I incorporated 4 ounces (113.4 g) of pure sesame oil. Even this lover of Oriental food couldn't pretend that the soap didn't reek of pungent sesame oil. It overpowered every other scent in the blend. I recommend the deodorized version. The spirulina powder colors the Sushi Bar a lovely sea green, and the millet seeds speckle the bar with an unusual grain.

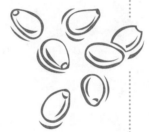

201 grams sodium hydroxide
1 pound 3 ounces (538.7 g) distilled water
1 pound 1 ounce (482 g) olive oil
1 pound (453.6 g) coconut oil
14 ounces (397 g) palm oil
4 ounces (113.4 g) sesame oil (deodorized)
2 tablespoons (30 ml) rice flour
1 tablespoon (15 ml) kelp powder
1 tablespoon (15 ml) ginseng root powder
1 teaspoon (5 ml) spirulina powder
1 tablespoon (15 ml) millet seeds
12 grams grapefruit seed extract (an optional preservative)
7 teaspoons (35 ml) Oriental blend of pure essential oils, optional
    (see chapter 6, pages 150–154)

## One essential oil blend option:

2¾ teaspoons (13.75 ml) sweet orange
2¾ teaspoons (13.75 ml) jasmine
1½ teaspoons (7 ml) vetiver

## Special Instructions
At the trace, add the rice flour, kelp powder, ginseng root powder, spirulina powder, and millet seeds. Then add the scent, if desired.

**Temperatures**

Fats and oils: 100°F (38°C)
Lye solution: 100°F (38°C)

Sodium Hydroxide Discount: 10%

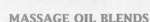

**MASSAGE OIL BLENDS**

Add 3½ teaspoons (17 ml) of
selected blend to each layer
of soap.

**Option A**
3 teaspoons (15 ml) lavender
2 teaspoons (10 ml) clary sage
2 teaspoons (10 ml) bergamot

**Option B**
2 teaspoons (10 ml) rosewood
2 teaspoons (10 ml) jasmine
1 teaspoon (5 ml) geranium
1½ teaspoons (7 ml) sweet orange
½ teaspoon (2 ml) patchouli

**Option C**
3 teaspoons (15 ml) lavender
3 teaspoons (15 ml) sandalwood
1 teaspoon (5 ml) geranium

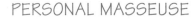
In our family, backrubs go back generations. My great-grandfather enjoyed a backrub as much as my youngest daughter does today. Years ago I saw a soap made with tapioca pearls designed by Barbara Bobo at Woodspirits, Ltd. I cannot recall the name of the bar, but I believe she created it with massage in mind. Tapioca pearls are derived from the root of the cassava plant; they are high in carbohydrates and are used to make pudding.

To Barbara's tapioca pearls I have added poppy seeds, for more texture and for the pretty appearance of black specks on a yellow background. I have also incorporated a variety of soothing, moisturizing massage oils. The massage layer of this bar contains the pearls and the seeds; the other layer is perfectly smooth for gentle lathering. After a week or so of use, the tapioca becomes mushy if it has been exposed to an excess of water. Use the pearls only to massage, relying upon the smooth side for lather. For a similar effect, experiment with wheat berries, millet seed, and mung beans.

**Bottom Layer**
1½ cups (375 ml) tapioca pearls
101 grams sodium hydroxide
9.5 ounces (269.3 g) distilled water
4.5 ounces (127.6 g) olive oil
2 ounces (56.7 g) wheat germ oil
2 ounces (56.7 g) sweet almond oil
8 ounces (226.8 g) coconut oil
2 ounces (56.7 g) cocoa butter
7 ounces (198.45 g) palm oil
1 tablespoon (15 ml) poppy seeds
6 grams grapefruit seed extract (an optional preservative)
3½ teaspoons (17 ml) pure essential oil or fragrance oil, optional (see box)

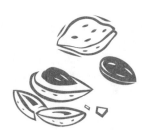

### Top Layer

101 grams sodium hydroxide
9.5 ounces (269.3 g) distilled water
4.5 ounces (127.6 g) olive oil
2 ounces (56.7 g) wheat germ oil
2 ounces (56.7 g) sweet almond oil
8 ounces (226.8 g) coconut oil
2 ounces (56.7 g) cocoa butter
7 ounces (198.45 g) palm oil
6 grams grapefruit seed extract (an optional preservative)
3½ teaspoons (17 ml) pure essential oil or fragrance oil, optional (see box)

## Special Instructions

**Bottom layer.** Pour the pearls evenly onto the waxed paper on the bottom of the mold. Prepare the soap as usual, using just the quantities listed for the bottom layer. At a full trace (wait for definite trailings) add the poppy seeds and any desired essential oil. Gently and evenly pour the soap mixture on top of the tapioca pearls. Cover the soap and insulate for three hours before adding the top layer.

**Top layer.** Prepare the soap as usual, using just the quantities listed for the top layer. Time this layer to be poured as soon as the bottom layer has cured for three hours. At the trace, pour the soap mixture over the hardened bottom layer. Re-cover the tray and insulate for another eighteen hours.

Cut finished bars immediately after the insulation period.

Cross-sectional view of the two layers: tapioca and poppy seed massage layer on bottom, smooth lathering layer on top.

## Temperatures

Fats and oils: 90–100°F (32–38°C)
Lye solution: 90–100°F (32–38°C)

Sodium Hydroxide Discount: 10%

### NOTE

Larger quantities of honey can replace a portion of the water (½–¾ cup). Add the sodium hydroxide to the water/honey mixture and proceed as usual. The active properties in the honey are destroyed by the lye, but the honey contributes richness, moisture, and color to the final bars.

# QUEEN OF THE NILE

Since everything we know about Cleopatra was written by her enemies, I'm not sure how we can know that she took milk baths. But the story has stuck, and even today we include milk and honey in skin-care preparations as soothing, emollient cleansers.

198 grams sodium hydroxide
12.8 ounces (362.9 g) distilled water
1 pound (453.6 g) olive oil
3.5 ounces (99.2 g) wheat germ oil
1 pound (453.6 g) coconut oil
14 ounces (397 g) palm oil
1.5 ounces (42.5 g) beeswax
½ cup (125 ml) oatmeal
6.4 ounces (181.4 g) buttermilk
12 grams grapefruit seed extract (an optional preservative)
10 teaspoons (50 ml) honey
7 teaspoons (35 ml) pure essential oil or fragrance oil, optional

### Special Instructions

Dissolve the sodium hydroxide into the 12.8 ounces (362.9 g) of water, stirring quickly to dissolve thoroughly. Combine the beeswax with the coconut and palm oils and heat until the beeswax is completely melted.

When the lye solution and the melted fats and oils come close to the desired soapmaking temperature, gently heat the milk to the same temperature. Whisking quickly and firmly with a stainless-steel whisk, add the buttermilk to the lye solution. Once it is well blended, immediately begin pouring the lye/milk mixture into the melted fats and oils, beating briskly and firmly from start to finish.

At the trace, incorporate the honey and the oatmeal, blending well before adding the essential or fragrance oil. Work quickly to avoid overly-thickened soap.

# THAI TO THE EAST

Thailand, with its Chinese and Indian influences, has synthesized all of my favorite herbs and spices into its own distinctive cuisine. Food presentation in this land of sweet gardenias and orchids and hibiscus is regarded as an art form — something to be appreciated beyond nourishment. Soap can do more than clean.

201 grams sodium hydroxide
13 ounces (368.5 g) distilled water
1 pound 5 ounces (595.4 g) olive oil
1 pound (453.6 g) coconut oil
14 ounces (397 g) palm oil
6 ounces (170 g) coconut milk
2 tablespoons (30 ml) rice flour
2 tablespoons (30 ml) tapioca flour
¼ teaspoon (1 ml) cardamom
2 tablespoons (30 ml) dried lemongrass
12 grams grapefruit seed extract (an optional preservative)
7 teaspoons (35 ml) pure essential oil or fragrance oil,
    optional (I like a lime blend)

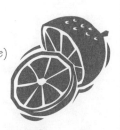

**Temperatures**

Fats and oils: 80–100°F (27–38°C)
Lye solution:   80–100°F (27–38°C)

Sodium Hydroxide Discount: 10%

**Special Instructions**
Prepare the soap as usual. Just before pouring the lye solution into the melted fats and oils, heat the coconut milk for ten seconds — only enough to melt it into liquid form. Do not let it get hot. Stirring continuously, add the lye to the fats and oils; then, without taking a break from the stirring, add the coconut milk to the soap mixture. Beat quickly and consistently from start to finish. At the trace, add the rice flour, tapioca flour, cardamom, and lemongrass. Finally, add any desired scent.

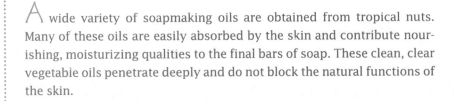

# NUTS ABOUT SOAP

**Temperatures**

Fats and oils: 80–95°F (27–35°C)
Lye solution: 80–95°F (27–35°C)

Sodium Hydroxide Discount: 10%

A wide variety of soapmaking oils are obtained from tropical nuts. Many of these oils are easily absorbed by the skin and contribute nourishing, moisturizing qualities to the final bars of soap. These clean, clear vegetable oils penetrate deeply and do not block the natural functions of the skin.

196 grams sodium hydroxide
13 ounces (368.5 g) distilled water
5 ounces (141.75 g) kukui nut oil
5 ounces (141.75 g) macadamia nut oil
5 ounces (141.75 g) hazelnut oil
4 ounces (113.4 g) jojoba oil
1 pound (453.6 g) coconut oil
2 ounces (56.7 g) cocoa butter
14 ounces (397 g) palm oil
6 ounces ( 170 g) coconut milk
½ cup (125 ml) ground almonds
12 grams grapefruit seed extract (an optional preservative)
7 teaspoons (35 ml) pure essential oil or fragrance oil, optional

**Special Instructions**

Prepare the soap as usual (remember that the solid cocoa butter is melted with the palm oil and the coconut oil). Just before pouring the lye solution into the melted fats and oils, heat the coconut milk for 10 seconds just to melt it into liquid form Do not let it get hot. Stirring continuously, add the lye to the fats and oils, and without taking a break from the stirring, add the coconut milk to the soap mixture. Beat the mixture quickly and consistently from start to finish. At trace, add the ground almonds. Finally, add any desired scent.

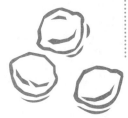

# NO-SEE-UMS SOAP

I have never lived in an area of the country without mosquitoes. As a camper, I've learned to accept their place in nature, though I try hard to limit the intrusion. This trooper is less charitable at bedtime, when the buzzing in my ear leaves me helplessly waiting for each new bite in the dark. Mosquitoes supposedly don't like a buildup of fatty oils on the skin, or the scent of certain strong essential oils. Take this bar into the woods with you and leave the sweet-smelling perfume at home.

201 grams sodium hydroxide
1 pound 3 ounces (538.7 g) distilled water
11 ounces (311.85 g) olive oil
3 ounces (85.05 g) castor oil
1 pound (453.6 g) coconut oil
1 pound 2 ounces (510.3 g) palm oil
3 ounces (85.05 g) shea butter
12 grams grapefruit seed extract (an optional preservative)
7 teaspoons (35 ml) pure essential oil blend or fragrance oil, optional
   (see box)

**Temperatures**

Fats and oils:  80–100°F (27–38°C)
Lye solution:   80–100°F (27–38°C)

Sodium Hydroxide Discount: 10%

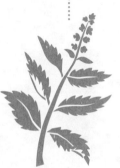

## INSECT REPELLENT OIL BLENDS

**Option A**
4 teaspoons (20 ml) lemongrass
1 teaspoon (5 ml) thyme
1 teaspoon (5 ml) peppermint
1 teaspoon (5 ml) lavender

**Option B**
2 teaspoons (10 ml) clove
2 teaspoons (10 ml) peppermint
3 teaspoons (15 ml) geranium

# DOWN THE GARDEN PATH

### Temperatures

Fats and oils  80–95°F (27–35°C)
Lye solution:  80–95°F (27–35°C)

Sodium Hydroxide Discount: 10%

New cities feel like home once you find your niche. Not long after I arrived in Memphis, my friend Urania shared her garden and the Memphis Herb Society with me. They all inspired me to get to work; the soil felt familiar and welcoming. "Build. . . Plant. . . Pray. . ." has always worked for me. The sooner I plant my garden, the sooner I feel at home.

I've added herbs to this soap in as many ways as possible — to the lye solution, the vegetable oils, the solid fats, and the final soap mixture. Any soapmaking formula will do; feel free to replace the hemp seed oil with another more accessible oil (and adjust the amount of sodium hydroxide). Add as few or as many different herbs as you'd like.

201 grams sodium hydroxide
1 pound 3 ounces (538.7 g)
  distilled water
9 ounces (255 g) olive oil
4 ounces (113.4 g) hemp seed oil
8 ounces (226.8 g) avocado oil
1 pound (453.6 g) coconut oil
14 ounces (397 g) palm oil

¼ cup (50 ml) wet comfrey leaves,
  dried or fresh, finely chopped
  and/or herbs for an herbal oil or
  an herbal infusion, see "Special
  Instructions," below
12 grams grapefruit seed extract
  (an optional preservative)
7 teaspoons (35 ml) pure essential
  oil or fragrance oil, optional

## Special Instructions

*Preparing the wet herbs.* Pour 1½ cups (375 ml) water over ¼ cup (50 ml) chopped comfrey leaves. Seal well and refrigerate for two to three days. Strain the herbs and squeeze out any excess water. Add the wet herbs at the trace, before you add the scent. Wet comfrey stays green for many weeks in the final bars; dried herbs always turn brown quickly.

*Preparing an herbal oil.* This can be done a couple of days before making the soap. (Herbal oils spoil quickly, so don't store for longer than a few days at room temperature.) Harvest a few handfuls of favorite herbs from the garden. Wash them lightly and pat as dry as possible. Warm the pre-measured olive and avocado oils (don't use the hemp seed oil until the day of soapmaking, to avoid premature spoilage) slightly and pour over the fresh herbs; stir gently for a few seconds. Cover tightly and let the herbal oil rest at room temperature for a day or so. Strain before using.

*Preparing an herbal infusion.* Once the sodium hydroxide is well dissolved in the water, add ½–1 cup (125–250 ml) of clean fresh or dried herbs. Stir occasionally to release the color from the herbs. Strain before adding the lye solution to the fats and oils.

## ESTHER'S ESTERS SHAMPOO BAR

The Tropical Shampoo Bar I included in *The Natural Soap Book* has been my favorite for years. Though the high percentage of castor oil and other unsaturated oils slows the hardening process, over time the soap becomes rock hard and the formula produces a rich, moisturizing lather. But I enjoy playing with new combinations, and the following recipe has been carefully designed to offer hardness without sacrificing conditioning qualities. By including slightly more saturated fats and increasing the percentage of sodium hydroxide, I have been able to keep the high percentage of castor oil — the ingredient most responsible for the dense, shaving cream–like lather. My feeling is that a shampoo bar without a meaningful percentage of castor oil is not appreciably different from a bar of soap. The soap can surely wash your hair, but a true shampoo bar more effectively conditions your hair and scalp.

**Temperatures**

Fats and oils: 100°F (38°C)
Lye solution: 100°F (38°C)

Sodium Hydroxide Discount: 10%

196 grams sodium hydroxide
1 pound 3 ounces (538.7 g)
   distilled water
3 ounces (85.05 g) avocado oil
4 ounces (113.4 g) wheat germ oil
9 ounces (255 g) castor oil
2 ounces (56.7 g) jojoba oil
1 pound (453.6 g) coconut oil

14 ounces (397 g) palm oil
1 ounce (28.35 g) shea butter
2 ounces (56.7 g) cocoa butter
12 grams grapefruit seed extract
   (an optional preservative)
7 teaspoons (35 g) pure essential
   oil or fragrance oil, optional

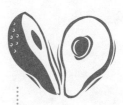

**Special Instructions**
Cut these bars immediately after the insulation period. Soon afterward, they become almost too hard to cut.

## Temperatures

Fats and oils: 80–100°F (27–38°C)
Lye solution: 80–100°F (27–38°C)

Sodium Hydroxide Discount: 10%

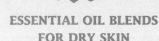

## ESSENTIAL OIL BLENDS FOR DRY SKIN

### Option A
4 teaspoons (20 ml) frankincense
3 teaspoons (15 ml) carrot seed

### Option B
3 teaspoons (15 ml) sandalwood
2 teaspoons (10 ml) geranium
1 teaspoon (5 ml) ylang-ylang
1 teaspoon (5 ml) rosewood

### Option C
2 teaspoons (10 ml) Roman chamomile
2 teaspoons (10 ml) geranium
1½ teaspoons (7 ml) rose
1½ teaspoons (7 ml) lavender

### Option D
3 teaspoons (15 ml) sandalwood
2 teaspoons (10 ml) rose
2 teaspoons (10 ml) Roman chamomile

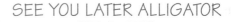

# SEE YOU LATER ALLIGATOR

The health of your skin relates in part to its ability to retain water. Unfortunately, heat, cold, pollution, ultraviolet rays, synthetic cosmetics, and poor diet inhibit the skin's ability to function normally. The result is sebaceous glands that no longer produce enough sebum — our bodies' natural source of fatty moisture — and, ultimately, dry skin. Water cannot take the place of sebum; instead, it evaporates from the surface of the skin, causing more dryness. Fatty acids from olive oil, avocado oil, sweet almond oil, wheat germ oil, and cocoa butter provide necessary moisture as well as a protective film that prevents moisture loss. This formula is designed to work cooperatively with lifestyle changes to restore the skin to a more normal state.

Note that hazelnut oil penetrates the skin easily and nourishes deeply. It is used to treat eczema because it stimulates the skin.

201 grams sodium hydroxide
1 pound 3 ounces (538.7 g) distilled water
6 ounces (170.1 g) hazelnut oil
5 ounces (141.75 g) avocado oil
6 ounces (170.1 g) wheat germ oil
4 ounces (113.4 g) sweet almond oil
1 pound (453.6 g) coconut oil
14 ounces (397 g) palm oil
12 grams grapefruit seed extract (an optional preservative)
7 teaspoons (35 ml) pure essential oil blend, optional (see box)

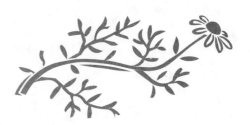

# DON'T SWEAT THE SMALL STUFF

Sweat doesn't smell, but the combination of bacteria and sweat does. How nice it would be if those deodorant stones worked for me, but they don't. I have yet to find a natural antiperspirant or deodorant as effective as the synthetic ones, and yet many persuasive articles describe some serious side effects: enlarged sweat glands, sebaceous cysts, pimples within the armpits, and even tumors. The more common stinging, itching, and rashes should put us on the alert.

This soap is designed as a deodorizing body bar, not a replacement for underarm deodorants, but it contributes to overall protection when used as a part of a more natural routine including frequent bathing, a healthful diet, and the use of herbal deodorants that fight bacteria.

**Temperatures**

Fats and oils: 80–100°F (27–38°C)
Lye solution: 80–100°F (27–38°C)

Sodium Hydroxide Discount: 10%

200 grams sodium hydroxide
1 pound 3 ounces (538.7 g) distilled water
8 ounces (226.8 g) calendula oil
9 ounces (255.15 g) wheat germ oil
4 ounces (113.4 g) castor oil
1 pound (453.6 g) coconut oil
14 ounces (397 g) palm oil
1 tablespoon (15 ml) vitamin E oil
2 tablespoons (30 ml) rice flour
2 tablespoons (30 ml) cornstarch
2 tablespoons (30 ml) aloe vera gel
1 teaspoon (5 ml) seaweed (spirulina, dulse, or Irish moss)
½ cup (125 ml) wet sage leaves (soaked in water for a few days and squeezed dry)
7 teaspoons (35 ml) deodorizing pure essential oils, optional (see box)

## Special Instructions

Add the vitamin E oil about halfway to the trace. Just before the trace, add the rice flour, cornstarch, seaweed, and damp sage leaves. At the trace, add the aloe vera gel and the essential oil.

## DEODORIZING ESSENTIAL OILS

**Option A**

3 teaspoons (15 ml) tea tree
1½ teaspoons (7 ml) thyme
1 teaspoon (5 ml) peppermint
1½ teaspoons (7 ml) clary sage

**Option B**

7 teaspoons (35 ml) anise seed

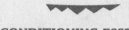

**CONDITIONING ESSENTIAL OIL BLEND**

2 teaspoons (10 ml) carrot
2 teaspoons (10 ml) parsley
3 teaspoons (15 ml) geranium

**Temperatures**

Fats and oils: 90–100°F (32–38°C)
Lye solution: 90–100°F (32–38°C)

Sodium Hydroxide Discount: 10%

This is a Julia Child–type recipe. It's not difficult, but it involves loads of ingredients and some fuss. Since the ingredients are costly, reserve this bar for special occasions. During the colder dry months, the conditioning formula soothes dry skin. It also makes a nice shampoo bar, though I often replace some of the unsaturated oil with more castor oil (and adjust the sodium hydroxide accordingly) for the thicker lather I like in a shampoo bar.

200 grams sodium hydroxide
1 pound 3 ounces (538.7 g)
   distilled water
3 ounces (85.05 g) castor oil
4 ounces (113.4 g) avocado oil
4 ounces (113.4 g) borage oil
4 ounces (113.4 g) evening
   primrose oil
4 ounces (113.4 g) sweet almond oil

2 ounces (56.7 g) sesame oil
1 pound (453.6 g) coconut oil
12 ounces (340.2 g) palm oil
1 ounce (28.35 g) shea butter
1 ounce (28.35 g) cocoa butter
12 grams grapefruit seed extract
   (an optional preservative)
7 teaspoons (35 ml) pure essential
   oil, optional (see box)

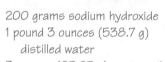

## TERRINE AUX TROIS LEGUMES

A few traditions are a given when my brother visits us here in Tennessee. We can count on his music and his famous fajitas, and before the week's end, Steve creates a new soap. This terrine was the product of one Thanksgiving visit; it reminds me of tricolored pasta. Another fun variation, Gift of the Sea, followed a month later when he spent Christmas with us. To convert the terrine into Gift of the Sea bars, use ⅔ teaspoon of ultramarine blue to color the first layer, white for the second, and the annatto for the third — top — layer. This is fresh and pretty, and designed to reflect the colors of summer at Cape Cod.

### First Layer

67 grams sodium hydroxide

6.3 ounces (178.6 g) distilled water

7 ounces (198 g) olive oil

5.5 ounces (156 g) coconut oil

4.5 ounces (128 g) palm oil

½ teaspoon (2.5 ml) powdered
natural chlorophyll

4 grams grapefruit seed extract
(optional preservative)

2¼ teaspoons (11.25 ml) pure
essential oil or fragrance oil,
optional

### Second Layer

67 grams sodium hydroxide

6.3 ounces (178.6 g) distilled water

7 ounces (198 g) olive oil

5.5 ounces (156 g) coconut oil

4.5 ounces (128 g) palm oil

4 grams grapefruit seed extract
(optional preservative)

2¼ teaspoons (11.25 ml) pure
essential oil or fragrance oil,
optional

### Third Layer

1 tablespoon plus 1 teaspoon
(20 ml) annatto seeds

67 grams sodium hydroxide

6.3 ounces (178.6 g) distilled water

7 ounces (198 g) olive oil

5.5 ounces (156 g) coconut oil

4.5 ounces (128 g) palm oil

4 grams grapefruit seed extract
(optional preservative)

2¼ teaspoons (11.25 ml) pure
essential oil or fragrance oil,
optional

### Special Instructions

Follow instructions for layered soap (see page 67). Be certain to stir each layer to a full trace — when the trailings just start to remain on the surface of the soap. Add the chlorophyll to the first layer immediately after adding the lye solution to the fats and oils. Before beginning the first layer, combine the annatto seeds for the third layer with ½ cup of olive oil and microwave on high for 30 seconds. Stir to release some color, cover, and stir periodically during the soapmaking process. To compensate for the annatto oil, weigh the required amount of olive oil for the third layer; then remove ½ cup and return to the bottle. Stir the annatto oil one final time, strain, and add to the olive oil.

**Note:** 1⅓ tablespoons of spirulina can be used in place of the powdered natural chlorophyll.

**Temperatures**

Fats and oils: 90–100°F (32–38°C)
Lye solution: 90–100°F (32–38°C)

Sodium Hydroxide Discount: 10%

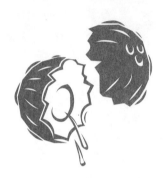

$M$y Thanksgiving candles gave me the idea for this color combination. The dark purple and the dark orange/yellow blend is a beautiful one — one of my favorites. (See Chapter 5, page 124, for another purple possibility.)

**Bottom Layer**

100.5 grams sodium hydroxide
9.5 ounces (269.3 g) distilled water
10.5 ounces (297.7 g) olive oil
8 ounces (226.8 g) coconut oil
7 ounces (198.5 g) palm oil

3 teaspoons (15 ml) ultramarine violet
6 grams grapefruit seed extract (optional preservative)
3.5 teaspoons (17.5 ml) pure essential oil or fragrance oil, optional

**Top Layer**

1 tablespoon plus 1 teaspoon (20 ml) annatto seeds
100.5 grams sodium hydroxide
9.5 ounces (269.3 g) distilled water
10.5 ounces (297.7 g) olive oil

8 ounces (226.8 g) coconut oil
7 ounces (198.5 g) palm oil
6 grams grapefruit seed extract (optional preservative)
3.5 teaspoons (15 ml) pure essential oil or fragrance oil, optional

**Special Instructions**

Follow instructions for layered soap (see page 67). Be certain to stir each layer to a full trace — when the trailings just begin to remain on the surface of the soap. Before beginning the bottom layer, combine the annatto seeds for the top layer with ½ cup of olive oil and microwave on high for 30 seconds. Stir to release some color, cover, and stir periodically during the soapmaking process.

Add the ultramarine violet to the hot lye solution of the bottom layer, or immediately after adding the lye solution to the fats and oils. Proceed as usual. For the top layer, weigh the required amount of olive oil; then remove ½ cup and return to the bottle to compensate for the annatto oil. Stir the annatto oil one final time, strain, and add to the olive oil.

# TAR BAR

**Temperatures**

Fats and oils: 100°F (38°C)
Lye solution: 100°F (38°C)

Sodium Hydroxide Discount: 10%

Tar is a dark, oily substance created as a by-product of the gases formed during the distillation of coal, wood, oils, and other organic matter. One kind of tar, pine tar, is obtained from the stumps of pine trees as a by-product of the paper industry. It is thought that this viscous, sticky material effectively treats a variety of skin diseases such as eczema, psoriasis, and dandruff. It is also considered antiseptic. I have used pine tar to treat and seal open wounds on chickens, and it is thought that pine tar soap, in combination with other treatment, helps to relieve the above skin conditions.

Pine tar soap has been around for a long time, but note the following warning: some people find pine tar to be a sensitizer, and the smell is pungent. I made a batch of pine tar soap and scented it with a strong blend of herbal oils, and I still had to let the batch cure in a remote part of the house. Today, sulfur is used to extract the crude oil from the pine wood while preparing paper, and the pine tar carries this sulfur smell. The scent diminishes over time, but this soap is not for everyone. I must say, however, that it has grown on me. Four ounces of pine tar can be added to a five-pound shampoo bar formula to treat dandruff. I exclude the grapefruit seed extract, as the pine tar does a fine job of preserving the soap.

201 grams sodium hydroxide
1 pound 3 ounces (538.7 g) distilled water
1 pound 5 ounces (595.4 g) olive oil
1 pound (453.6 g) coconut oil
14 ounces (397 g) palm oil
4 ounces (113.4 g) pine tar
7 teaspoons (35 ml) pure essential oil or fragrance oil, optional

## Special Instructions

Though pine tar can be added at trace if the soapmaker works quickly to ensure no lumps, I add the pine tar to the melted fats and oils immediately before adding the lye solution. The pine tar speeds up saponification, so be ready to add essential oils and pour within two to five minutes.

## Temperatures

Fats and oils: 100°F (38°C)
Lye solution: 100°F (38°C)

Sodium Hydroxide Discount: 0%

# BLOWIN' IN THE WIND LAUNDRY SOAP

Homemade laundry soap is a treat. Its clean, sweet smell is a step backward in the right direction. In contrast to the highly synthetic laundry soap available at the supermarket, this version contains only pure, basic ingredients — nothing more. The borax is thought to quicken the sudsing action, retard the formation of mildew, and soften water. The vinegar softens the clothes and keeps them colorfast. The baking soda, the vinegar, and the borax freshen the clothes by ridding them of perspiration and odors.

Detergents are effective in soft and hard water and contain enzymes that chemically dissolve a wide range of stains. Homemade soap loses stain contests, but it does a beautiful job cleaning more average loads of dirty laundry. I keep a bottle of the spray-and-wash type laundry treatments handy for blood, grass, and tomato sauce, but this old-fashioned laundry soap formula leaves towels and clothing clean and fresh after normal wear and tear. About 1 cup of soap cleans an average load of laundry; 1½–1¾ cups may be needed for heavy-duty cleaning.

Once they are in bar form, Laundry Bars can be shredded and heated in water to produce a liquid or solid-gel version for the washing machine. Recipes for the gel and liquid versions follow.

220 grams sodium hydroxide
19 ounces (538.65 g) distilled water
  minus ¾ cup (175 ml), to be used as
  described in Special Instructions
4 tablespoons (60 ml) borax
½ tablespoon (7.5 ml) salt
1 tablespoon (15 ml) sugar
2 tablespoons (30 ml) ammonia,
  optional

21 ounces (595.35 g) coconut oil
24 ounces (680.4 g) vegetable
  shortening
24 ounces (680.4 g) palm oil
3–4 tablespoons (45–60 ml)
  baking soda, sifted through
  fine-mesh strainer

**Special Instructions**
Immediately after thoroughly dissolving the sodium hydroxide in the water, dissolve the borax into the lye solution, stirring until well

incorporated. Bring the ¾ cup (175 ml) reserved water nearly to a boil, and then add the salt and sugar; when both have dissolved, add the ammonia and blend well. When the fats and oils and the lye solution reach the desired soapmaking temperatures, warm the salt/sugar/ammonia solution to 100°F. Add the lye solution to the fats and oils, stirring briskly and continuously. Immediately add the salt/sugar/ammonia solution and continue a brisk, regular stir. As the soap mixture approaches the trace, add the baking soda and blend well. (Adding the baking soda at the trace does not allow enough stirring time for a more complete incorporation of the baking soda.)

**Note:** The baking soda can be mixed with just enough water to dissolve the baking soda before adding the soda water to the still-hot lye/borax solution. I prefer to add the baking soda a few minutes before trace. A few tiny specks of unincorporated baking soda does not affect the quality of the soap.

## OTHER USES

This laundry soap is also an excellent general purpose cleaner. Both the gel and the liquid soap can be used to clean floors, counters, walls, and appliances inexpensively.

### Making Laundry Gel

As soon as possible after the laundry soap's eighteen-hour insulation period, cut it into large bars, without worrying about form. Within the next few hours — before they become too hard — shred the bars using a hand-held cheese shredder. This is easy when the bars are fresh and firm but not yet rock hard.

Place the soap shreds into a large stockpot and cover with 8 cups (2 liters) of clean water. Bring the water to a boil, turn the heat to medium-low, and let the mixture simmer for ten minutes. Pour it into a heat-proof container and allow it to cool to room temperature before covering tightly. Within a day or so, the soap mixture will solidify into a gel that melts perfectly into a load of laundry — even a load washed with cold water.

### Making Liquid Laundry Soap

Follow the above instructions for laundry gel, but add 2 cups (500 ml) vinegar to the 8 cups (2 liters) water in the stockpot. This formula creates a rich, white liquid with the softening properties of vinegar. If a slight separation occurs over time, stir the mixture before each use.

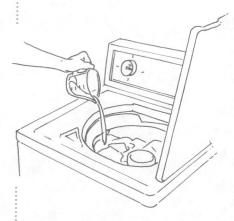

# TALL ORDER

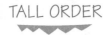

**Temperatures**

Fats and oils: 90–100°F (32–38°C)
Lye solution: 90–100°F (32–38°C)

Sodium Hydroxide Discount: 8%

Tall oil, known as liquid rosin, is a mixture of fatty acids and resin obtained as a by-product of the wood pulp industry. After processing, the black crude oil becomes lighter and clear with a pleasant smell. With 50–60 percent fatty acids, tall oil saponifies readily and is used to make liquid and solid soap and detergent. Tall oil is known to produce a generous soap lather, but like pine tar, it can be a mild irritant for sensitive individuals. I reserve this bar for household cleaning and laundry.

204 grams sodium hydroxide
1 pound 3 ounces (538.7 g) distilled water
10 ounces (283.5 g) tall oil
11 ounces (311.85 g) olive oil
1 pound (453.6 g) coconut oil
14 ounces (397 g) palm oil
12 grams grapefruit seed extract (optional preservative)
7 teaspoons (35 ml) pure essential oil or fragrance oil, optional

**Special Instructions**

Tall oil saponifies more quickly than any other oil I've worked with, turning the soap mixture into a wonderfully smooth cream before the soap can be poured. The process is almost instantaneous, even when the tall oil accounts for only a small percentage of the total fats and oils. Add scent to the traced soap; then spread as evenly as possible with a spatula. The final bars are rich and creamy looking with a generous lather. Trim the soap after the eighteen-hour insulation period.

# GUM ROZ'N BARS

Rosin has been added to opaque soap for its lathering qualities and to transparent soap for its transparency. Rosin contributes a quick, full, fluffy lather even in small percentages. Unlike some other rosins, gum rosin does not darken the soap. If it is easily accessible, add rosin to laundry soap formulas for the fullest lather. Note that any rosin can cause contact dermatitis in sensitive individuals.

201 grams sodium hydroxide
1 pound 3 ounces (538.7 g) distilled water
1 pound (453.6 g) coconut oil
14 ounces (396.9 g) palm oil
4 ounces (113.4 g) gum rosin
1 pound 5 ounces (595.4 g) olive oil
12 teaspoons (60 ml) grapefruit seed extract (optional preservative)
7 teaspoons (35 ml) pure essential oil or fragrance oil, optional

**Special Instructions**

Heat the rosin along with the coconut oil and the palm oil to 180°F (82°C) to completely melt the rosin. Add the olive oil and cool the mixture to 100°F (38°C). Cold-process rosin soap can be slightly grainy, so be sure to beat the mixture well.

**Temperatures**

Fats and oils: 100°F (38°C)
Lye solution: 90°F (32°C)

Sodium Hydroxide Discount: 5%

# NATIVE BLEND MOISTURIZING CREAM

*Makes about eleven 4-ounce (113 g) jars*

I tuck my cream formulas into the book as a small gift. Over the last few years, I have received letters from people frustrated by natural cream formulations. Most natural creams are beeswax emulsions, combinations of vegetable oils, water, beeswax, and borax (plus any variety of nutrients). The beeswax and borax unite the incompatible ingredients — the water and the oils. Beeswax emulsions tend to be much thicker than commercial creams that rely upon synthetic chemicals for a thinner consistency. After much trial and error, I found my way to lighter beeswax emulsions.

It is the correct balance of oils, beeswax, borax, and water that determines the texture of a natural cream; too much beeswax, saturated fats, and borax makes the cream too thick, and too much water and oil causes separation. For a looser cream, replace a small portion of the beeswax and borax with an equal amount of water, noting that you ride a fine line between separation and paste. For a slightly more dense cream, replace a small portion of the water or the oil with more beeswax, borax, and saturated fats, like shea or cocoa butter. I stress the need to make changes in small increments (20–30 grams at a time) to not radically upset the balance.

Once the basic formula is perfectly balanced, variation is simple and fun. You can incorporate fun nutrients like herbal infusions, aloe vera gel, tea tree oil, seaweed, herbs, honey, goat's milk, buttermilk, rosewater, or cucumber juice, and substitute oils like rosa mosqueta rose hip seed, calendula, borage, and macadamia nut for any portion of the listed oils. Just be careful to replace one consistency for another comparable one: liquid for liquid, oil for oil, and dense solid for dense solid. My cream is highly concentrated, so dab it on lightly and blend well.

### Selecting a Formulation

Choose the formulation that produces the most desirable texture; they are not listed in order of preference. Formulation #1, "Light & Loose," is for those who prefer more of a lotion. The addition of any more liquid is likely to cause separation, for I have pushed this blend to its limit in an effort to produce a thinner, yet rich, cream. Formulation #2, "Light Soufflé," is as smooth and light as #1, but it holds its form like an airy soufflé. Formulation #3, "Firm Mousse," is firmer than the soufflé — more like a whipped mousse. Though slightly grainy, this cream is light and airy and melts easily into the skin. Formulation #4, "Firm & Creamy," is perfectly creamy, with a slightly heavier consistency than the other three variations. I am not a fan of buttery salves, but any of these formulations can be easily converted into more dense mixtures; to do so, replace a portion of the water and the liquid vegetable oils with saturated fats and beeswax, and slightly more borax.

Finally, for a little fun, color the cream with a few of the natural colorants in chapter 5. For whiter cream, replace the wheat germ oil with clear vegetable oils like olive, sweet almond, castor, kukui nut, avocado, or apricot kernel. The wheat germ oil produces a warm yellow tone; increase the percentage of it for a deeper shade (decreasing another oil by an equal percentage). Occasionally, I make a warm brown cream (it does not bleed) using vanilla fragrance oil or Peru balsam essential oil. If desired, you can color cream blue, green, violet, pink, and orange to match your soaps.

**Instructions**

Measure the essential or fragrance oil and set aside in a tightly sealed container. Use two saucepans — one for the oil mixture and one for the water mixture. Heat both mixtures to 165°F (74°C). Be sure that the borax dissolves completely into the water and that the beeswax fully melts from the heat of the oils. Monitor the temperature to avoid overheating.

Pour the oil mixture into the mixing bowl. Using a freestanding electric mixer with a splash-guard, and set at the lowest

| INGREDIENTS | FORMULATIONS (IN GRAMS) | | | |
|---|---|---|---|---|
| | Light & Loose | Light Soufflé | Firm Mousse | Firm & Creamy |
| **Oil Phase** | | | | |
| olive oil | 310 | 275 | 250 | 325 |
| sweet almond oil | 50 | 50 | 50 | 50 |
| wheat germ oil | 25 | 25 | 25 | 25 |
| jojoba oil | 35 | 35 | 50 | 40 |
| shea butter | 15 | 15 | 10 | 10 |
| castor oil | 15 | 15 | 20 | — |
| cocoa butter | — | 15 | 20 | — |
| beeswax | 75 | 75 | 100 | 75 |
| grapefruit seed extract | 10 | 10 | — | — |
| **Water Phase** | | | | |
| distilled water | 433.5 | 413.5 | 440 | 443.5 |
| borax | 10 | 10 | 10 | 10 |
| vegetable glycerin | 15 | 15 | 15 | 15 |
| Essential Oil or Fragrance Oil | 6 | 6 | 5 | 6 |

speed, slowly drizzle the water mixture into the oils. Continue to blend on low until the mixture thickens slightly, scraping any solid or liquid buildup that clings to the sides of the bowl back into the cream. When it has thickened just enough to tolerate a faster stir without splashing wildly, increase the mixer speed to setting 2 (the cream is still pretty watery). When it thickens further (this takes about ten to fifteen minutes), scrape the sides of the bowl again and increase the speed to setting 3. Continue beating until cream is the consistency of mayonnaise.

Once the mixture is uniform and has begun to cool (the mixing bowl should feel not hotter than lukewarm), add the essential oil and continue beating to fully incorporate the scent. At this point of production, a fast stir (setting 3 or 4) is critical for a perfectly creamy blend.

When the cream is smooth and cold, pour into jars, rewhipping cream in bowl periodically with a whisk to ensure mixture is uniform. To avoid separation in more liquid formulas, first pour into a covered container, allow to rest for at least six hours, and rewhip in mixer at fast speed just until it forms rich, soft peaks, then spoon into jars.

## NOTE

When I first made cream years ago, I was not biased toward natural preservatives, though I'd gone to great lengths to wrestle natural ingredients into a stable formulation. I used methyl paraben (for the water phase) and propyl paraben (for the oil phase) after some research suggested that these were two safe synthetic preservatives, especially in such small percentages (.1 percent methyl paraben — 1 gram into the formulations — and .05 percent propyl paraben — ½ gram into the formulations). A fatty cream needs protection to delay spoilage, but there are other options. Grapefruit seed extract, the natural preservative I include in my soap formulas, offers limited protection to cream; though the parabens protect for years, grapefruit seed extract extends shelf life for enough months to satisfy most demands. Note that grapefruit seed extract adds more liquid to the blend, so when adding it to your favorite formulations, reduce the percentage of water to avoid separation. Also, consider skipping a preservative when making small batches that can be used within a couple of months. Again, note that removing grapefruit seed extract from a formula reduces the liquid for a somewhat firmer cream; add more water to compensate for the loss if a looser cream is desired. Finally, refrigeration is always an option, but it stiffens the cream.

# NATIVE BLEND LIP BALM
*Makes 30 jars*

A natural lip balm is simple to make and much more effective than the petrolatum-based lip balms typically found in stores. Though petrolatum (petroleum jelly) offers some immediate relief from chapping, continued use actually dries lips and skin further. Moisturizing vegetable oils, vegetable glycerin, and beeswax soothe and soften lips as they lay a protective barrier to guard against moisture loss and environmental attack.

I prefer a softer consistency to the rock-hard beeswax balms, so I incorporate a high percentage of oils and only enough beeswax to firm the mixture. Adjust the ratios to accommodate your preference. I do not include a preservative; jojoba oil, castor oil, wheat germ oil, beeswax, and vegetable glycerin do not deteriorate quickly, and wheat germ oil has antioxidant properties to protect the more vulnerable oils. Since the lip balm lasts for months, unrefrigerated, I do not bother with grapefruit seed extract, which has an unpleasant taste. Only use the most mild, food-grade essential oils for scent (no fragrance oils and no irritating essential oils). Feel free to cut back the formula for smaller batches.

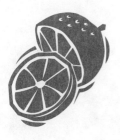

30 grams (1 ounce) *coconut oil*
80 grams (2.8 ounces) *castor oil*
60 grams (2.1 ounces) *jojoba oil*
20 grams (.7 ounce) *beeswax*
30 grams (1 ounce) *wheat germ oil*

40 grams (1.4 ounces) *vegetable glycerin*
1 teaspoon (5 ml) *pure essential oil (I like sweet orange or grapefruit)*

In a small heavy-duty saucepan over low heat, combine all of the ingredients except for the pure essential oil and heat just until the beeswax melts. Remove from heat and add the pure essential oil. Pour into lip balm jars, restirring the mixture after pouring a few jars to be sure that the essential oil and the vegetable glycerin are in solution. (These two ingredients are water-soluble and do not perfectly blend with the oils.)

# CHAPTER 2
## Special Techniques

I never thought of soap as a medium until I began experimenting with shape, color, and texture. Now I see soapmaking as another opportunity for art and function to work cooperatively. Like a blank canvas, a batch of white soap begs for a splash of color. Smooth soap can be made scratchy. Varied shapes introduce personality.

I think that a pure bar of soap with a creamy color, a silky texture, and a wholesome scent is beautiful. It needs no embellishment. And yet I cannot keep from tinkering with the endless possibilities for variation. Though we all make fundamentally similar soap, our soaps still somehow reflect our unique natures. One soap is brightly colored, another is muted. One bar is filled with herbs and grains, another is solid and smooth. One bar makes an environmental statement, another is playful.

In this chapter, I present nine special techniques that you can use — as long as you can meet a few conditions. For instance, marbling is most successful if soapmaking temperatures are at least 90°F (32°C), and imprinting works best with soapmaking formulas that contain a high percentage of saturated fats and oils. Once you have a good understanding of various fats and oils and the characteristics each produces in your final bars of soap, you can transform your favorite soapmaking formulas by using them to create new designs.

## LIQUID SOAP

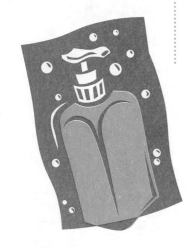

Just a couple of months ago, I received a letter from a man asking me how to make a natural liquid soap in the home. I had always been told that liquid soap required the addition of various synthetics to produce a consistency that could be pumped smoothly through a dispenser, and this is the information I passed along. I have since learned that this isn't the whole truth.

Homemade liquid soap is less than ideal, but I love it and am willing to scale down my expectations when my reward is, once again, the ability to control my skin-care products and produce them inexpensively. The following formulas require some fuss — some straining and dilution is involved — but the final results are nice. Also, the pump may need a periodic rinse with hot water for clog-free pumping. But the soap is rich and gentle; it contains no synthetic materials, other than the potassium hydroxide used to make most liquid soap; it is economical; and I can scent (or not scent) it as I please.

## Liquid Soap Production

Liquid soaps are usually potassium soaps that have been diluted with varying proportions of water. (Potassium soaps are made with potassium hydroxide as opposed to sodium soaps, which are made with sodium hydroxide.) The vegetable oils of choice are coconut oil and palm kernel oil, since the high–lauric acid oils are the ones that contribute a fluffy lather. Oils such as olive, castor, peanut, soy, and safflower do not produce much lather and therefore produce unexciting liquid soap, though they can be included as minority oils to contribute emollience. Liquid soap is fully saponified, because any unsaponified fats and oils will inhibit lather and consistency.

Though liquid soap can be produced using only coconut oil, potassium hydroxide, and water — and nothing else — many companies add alcohol and other clarifiers to make the soap completely transparent, along with synthetic chemicals to perfect the consistency. The soap is typically either cooked for hours or processed under pressure in an enclosed vessel. These processes and the required raw materials are not accessible to the home soapmaker, but a version of industrial soap can still be easily prepared in the kitchen.

Industrially, liquid soap is cooked for eight to twenty-four hours, or until transparency is achieved, with water added periodically to replace the evaporated portion. This process requires mechanized equipment to heat and stir the soap during all of these hours. Even industrial soapmaking involves some imprecision. Some batches

**Emollience**

The softening and soothing of the skin produced as substances called emollients spread onto the skin, acting as a barrier against moisture loss to the environment. (Insufficient moisture in the layers of skin called the stratum corneum causes dry skin.)

solidify and others remain fluid, depending upon the degree of evaporation — the ratio of soap to water — and a technician must monitor each batch and add water, much the way a chef adjusts a slow-cooking tomato sauce.

Potassium soap is much less temperamental than its sodium counterpart. It changes state — from liquid to solid and back to liquid — without much disturbance, and it can tolerate high temperatures without curdling. This margin for error allows the home soapmaker to tweak it until just the right consistency is achieved. The industrial soapmaker adds water periodically as the soap cooks to its finished state. The hours of hot processing produce perfect transparency.

By forfeiting transparency, however, I can shave twenty-three and a half hours off the processing time. My version of liquid soap is crude, but it works and it is easy. I make the soap in two phases. The first phase of production is exact and doesn't take long: I create a soap base, not worrying a bit at this point about the perfect consistency, focusing instead upon perfect saponification and the full incorporation of ingredients. During the second phase the next day, I add water to achieve my desired consistency.

Some liquid soaps are watery, and others are thicker. Their consistencies are the direct result of the percentage of soap in relation to the percentage of water. The soap base can account for between 15 and 40 percent of the liquid soap. My formulas incorporate between 35 and 40 percent soap and 60 and 65 percent water for a soap with more body. I'm not fond of the more watery liquid soap often found in public rest rooms.

### CAUTION

The "cooking" of liquid soap usually leaves it completely saponified and safe for use. I often use it immediately after the second phase of production. If the soap feels at all harsh just after the twenty-four hour rest period (test the lather of a small dab of soap and a little warm water), let the solid base cure for another week or two before proceeding with the second phase.

# SEAFARER'S SOAP

The most effective liquid soap is one made with 100 percent coconut oil or palm kernel oil. These high–lauric acid oils produce a superior lather, though they can be sensitizers for some people. Seafarer's Soap is the simplest of the three liquid soap formulas in this book; it includes only coconut oil, potassium hydroxide, and water.

29.5 grams (1 ounce) potassium hydroxide, flake or pellet
72 grams (2.5 ounces) distilled water
110 grams (3.8 ounces) 76°F (24.4°C) coconut oil, not hydrogenated
70 grams (2.5 ounces) distilled water
½ teaspoon (2 ml) pure essential oil or fragrance oil, optional

**1.** Dissolve the potassium hydroxide into the 72 g (2.5 ounces) water and set aside to cool to between 80°F and 100°F (27°C and 38°C).

**2.** When the potassium hydroxide solution has cooled sufficiently, heat the coconut oil and the 70 g (2.5 ounces) of water together in a heavy-bottomed saucepan to 180°F (82°C). The globules of oil will remain suspended in the water until the next step.

**3.** Off the heat, drizzle the potassium hydroxide solution into the oils and water, and gently stir to blend.

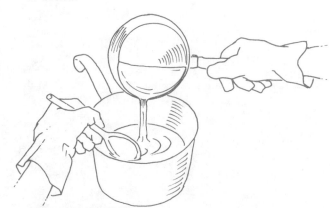

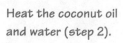
Heat the coconut oil and water (step 2).

Drizzle the potassium hydroxide solution into oils (step 3).

**4.** Place the pan back on the stove on a setting of low or medium-low (setting of 2 or 3) until the mixture creeps back up toward 180°F (82°C), stirring continuously but gently to create a uniform mixture. At first, the mixture looks like water shimmering with unsaponified oils, but after ten to fifteen minutes it will gradually become thick and uniform. Do not allow the temperature of the soap to exceed 180°F (82°C) or fall below 160°F (71°C); remove the pan from heat occasionally and return to the stove as needed.

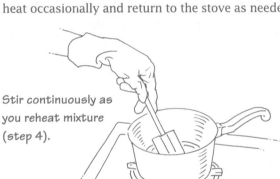

Stir continuously as you reheat mixture (step 4).

**5.** After fifteen minutes or so, the mixture is still liquid but gel-like, and on its way to becoming solid gel. Before it hardens too much, pour it into a heat-resistant container to solidify and cool. Leave for twenty-four hours.

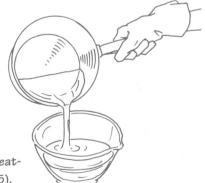

Pour gel-like mixture into heat-resistant container (step 5).

**6.** After the twenty-four hour wait or within the next eight to twelve weeks, the base can be converted to liquid soap. To do this, scoop half of the soap (save the other half until you need to make more soap) into a heavy-bottomed saucepan and add ½ cup (125 ml) water. With the stove set at medium-low, heat the soap and water without ever stirring. Stirring works up a lather, something undesirable at this stage. Instead heat slowly while scrunching the soap into the hot water, until the soap and water have blended into a uniform liquid soap.

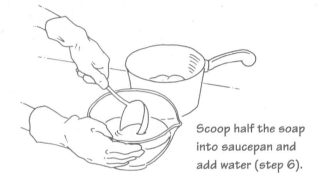

Scoop half the soap into saucepan and add water (step 6).

Heat slowly while scrunching the soap into the water.

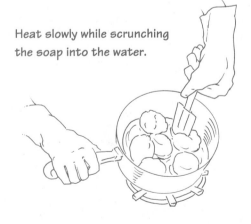

**7.** Using a fine-mesh strainer, strain the soap into a glass measuring cup to remove any traces of lather or undissolved soap. Then pour into a liquid soap dispenser.

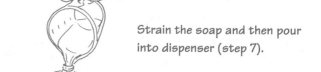

*Strain the soap and then pour into dispenser (step 7).*

## TRANSLUCENT GLYCERIN SOAP

This liquid soap formula is designed for people who react to pure coconut oil soap and need the added castor oil and glycerin for emollience.

34 grams (1.2 ounces) potassium
   hydroxide, flake or pellet
71 grams (2.5 ounces) distilled water
107.7 grams (3.8 ounces) coconut
   oil, not hydrogenated

22 grams (.77 ounces) castor oil
74 grams (2.6 ounces) distilled water
22 grams (.77 ounces) vegetable glycerin
½ teaspoon (2 ml) pure essential oil
   or fragrance oil, optional

**1.** Dissolve the potassium hydroxide into the 71 g (2.5 ounces) water and set aside to cool to between 80°F and 100°F (27°C and 38°C).
**2.** When the potassium hydroxide solution has cooled sufficiently, heat the coconut and castor oils and the 74 g (2.6 ounces) of water together in a heavy-bottomed saucepan to 180°F (82°C).
**3.** Place the pan back on the burner at a setting of 3 (medium-low) and continue to stir slowly and gently until soap begins to form. By the time the soap reaches 180°F (82°C), the mixture should be thickening slightly. At this temperature, add the 160–180°F (71–82°C) vegetable glycerin and gently and slowly incorporate it into the soap mixture.
**4.** Pour well-blended mixture into a heat-resistant container to cool. After ten minutes, add the essential oil, stirring ever-so-gently. Allow to cool without stirring again for thirty minutes, then pour into a container with a tight-fitting lid. (If a film formed on surface of the soap, pour through a fine-mesh strainer.) Continue as described in Seafarer's Soap (see step 6, page 60).

# PEARLESCENT LIQUID SOAP

This formula is processed differently than are the other two liquid soap recipes. The soap base is prepared more as an opaque soap is, though with less water, and the additives are whipped into the soap as it cools. The result is a thick white soap.

15 ml (1 tablespoon) sugar
91 grams (3.2 ounces) distilled water, boiling
34 grams (1.2 ounces) potassium hydroxide, flake or pellet
30 grams (1.05 ounces) distilled water
110 grams (3.8 ounces) coconut oil
22 grams (.77 ounces) castor oil
22 grams (.77 ounces) vegetable glycerin
½ teaspoon (2 ml) pure essential oil or fragrance oil, optional

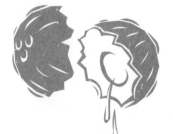

**1.** Dissolve the sugar into the 91 g (3.2 ounces) of boiling water. Cover and set aside.

**2.** Dissolve the potassium hydroxide into the 30 g (1.05 ounces) of water and set aside.

**3.** Heat the coconut oil and castor oil over low heat until the coconut oil melts. Remove the pan from the heat and allow the oils and the potassium hydroxide solution to cool for five more minutes.

**4.** Drizzle the potassium hydroxide solution into the oils, whisking continuously with a stainless-steel whisk until the mixture traces. Once it does, place the pan back on the stove, set on medium-low, and heat the soap to 120°F (49°C). Add the vegetable glycerin to the warm soap, blending well.

**5.** Reheat the sugar solution quickly to around 140–150°F (60–65.5°C).

**6.** Add the hot sugar solution to the soap, gently blending the mixture. Heat to 160°F (71°C); then pour the soap into a heat-resistant glass pitcher. Some stable lather will float on the surface of the mixture, but it will eventually be incorporated. Allow the soap to rest for ten minutes; then whisk the separated mixture well before placing the bowl in the refrigerator.

**7.** Whisk the refrigerated mixture every five to ten minutes until it is cool and well blended. Refrigeration is no longer necessary once the soap mixture stops separating between stirrings. Pour into a container and cover.

**8.** A day later, pour the soap into a heavy-bottomed saucepan and add a few tablespoons of water (as little as necessary for your desired consistency). Over medium-low heat, warm the soap slightly; then gently blend the soap and water to your desired consistency. Add the essential oil and pour into a liquid soap dispenser.

## MARBLING SOAP

I love the contrast of bright swirls of color on a white background. Though I make more solid-color bars than marbled ones, this technique is a favorite — and one well worth the fuss.

It's a fuss because at the most harried moment of the soapmaking process, marbling requires perfect orchestration. Once you add scent to soap, the mixture becomes a ticking time bomb ready at any moment to begin setting up. And it is after you add the scent that you must begin to draw color into the soap for marbling.

But with a little practice and few distractions, you can get the hang of this technique. I use midrange soapmaking temperatures (90–100°F [32–38°C]) for marbled batches. The lowest and highest soapmaking temperatures produce more reactive soap mixtures that thicken too quickly — before I've had a chance to thoroughly marble the contrasting color. The ideal mixture for marbling is one that remains fluid until both colors have been artistically blended, yet thick enough that separation is not of concern.

## Making Marbled Soap

You can produce a lovely marbled soap using any of your favorite soap formulas and the colorants of your choice (see chapter 5).

**1.** Choose two (or more) contrasting colors for the two soap mixtures — one for the base soap and one for the contrasting soap. (I like to use two-thirds base-color soap and one-third contrasting-color soap for a more striking effect.) Note that you achieve the marbling by removing a portion of the base soap mixture, coloring it, then swirling this colored soap into the base soap. Of course, two completely different batches of soap can be marbled into one another, but I usually use one batch.

**2.** Prepare your marbling utensils and ingredients and have them waiting by the soap mold for the big moment: colorant carefully measured into a bowl, whisk, measuring cup, plate, spatula (or knife), and essential oil.

**3.** Prepare soap according to the directions for your particular formula. When a *light* trace has been achieved, use a measuring cup to transfer about one-third (or however much you prefer) of the base soap to the bowl or large (6-cup) glass measuring cup containing the colorant. Work quickly and firmly to whisk the colorant evenly into the soap.

**4.** Still working swiftly, scent the base soap (if desired). Stir the mixture to be sure it is uniform and smooth; then pour it into the soap mold.

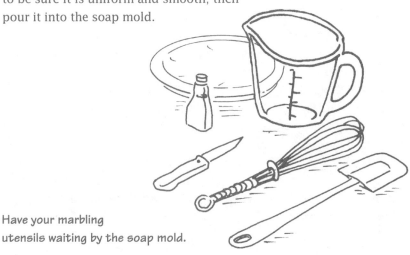

**Have your marbling utensils waiting by the soap mold.**

**5.** Scent the smaller, contrasting mixture (if desired; I usually don't), and pour the mixture in parallel lines across and down the base soap from a few inches above the soap mold, to force the soap down into the soap, not just onto the surface. How many lines you make depends upon the size of your soap mold, but aim for a line every 2–3 inches (5–7.6 cm) both lengthwise and crosswise.

**6.** Stand a spatula, knife, or honey drizzle upright at one corner of the soap tray, through to the waxed paper (if using a knife, avoid contact with the paper). Using a zigzag motion (in a diagonal pattern to the oppo-site corner), marble the contrasting color through the base color, crossing the "pour lines" at varying angles. Stand the spatula at one of the two corners, and repeat the step just described. Save a little of the contrasting soap to drizzle here and there on the surface; otherwise, the tops of the bars will not have enough of the marbled, contrasting color.

If you do not work quickly enough, the base color will begin to set up before you have marbled the contrasting color. Though the base is soft enough to weave the utensil through, both soap colors will form mounds during the marbling process. The surface will end up looking frosting like instead of being perfectly flat and smooth. Fortunately, this is not really a problem. Once the soap has hardened, you can level the ridges and valleys by slicing down to a level layer. The quality of the soap will not be affected.

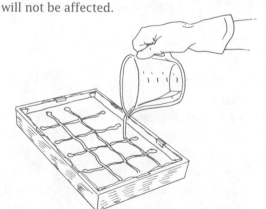

Pour lines of contrasting soap across top of base soap (step 5).

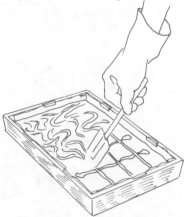

Make a zigzag motion across entire tray (step 6).

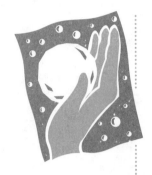

# SOAP BALLS

Soap balls can be made from fresher, still-somewhat-soft soap, or from shredded strips of soap.

## From Fresh Soap

To make soap balls from fresh soap, allow your soap to stay in the mold for a day or so, until it is firm to the touch but not rock hard. Cut into bars, but don't be concerned with symmetry. Remove the bars from the mold and slice off any residue on the surface. Roll each bar into a tightly compacted ball using the innermost portion of your palms, squeezing out any pockets of air. Allow the soap balls to rest on a dry, porous surface. Periodically, over the next few days, repeat the squeezing process a few times to smooth any large imperfections. I find the irregularities more interesting than perfect roundness; if you agree, leave some lumps and bumps for texture.

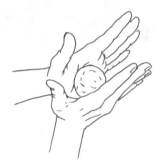

Roll each soap bar firmly into a compact ball between the palms of your hands.

## From Shredded Soap

Shredded soap can be kneaded with a little water to form another kind of soap ball. I like to use the plastic (flexible) moister shreds from one- to three-week-old soap. Cut the bars into manageable chunks and shred them in a food processor or with a hand shredder. Once you have a pile of shredded soap, add a tablespoon (15 ml) of water and a few drops of essential oil (if the soap is scented, only use water) for every cup (250 ml) of shredded soap, and knead the mixture until the water is fully incorporated. Make whatever slight adjustments you need until the mixture is smooth and firm and plastic. If the mixture is sticky, add more soap shreds; if it is dry, add a few drops of water at a time until you reach your desired consistency. Roll into compact balls, as described above.

## Variation

You can vary soap balls by incorporating different colors and textures of soap. Into mostly dark soap shreds, scatter a few shreds of lightly colored soap. Into a white base, add a variety of colored shreds for a confetti look. When soap balls are made with fresher, more plastic shreds, you can roll the outsides of the balls in finely shredded soap; these soap balls look like they are coated with shredded coconut.

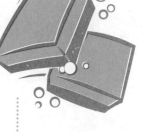

## LAYERING SOAP

Layering is easy once you get the hang of it and the effect can be striking. Just as it sounds, layering is achieved by pouring layers of soap on top of one another.

### Making Layered Soap

**1.** Plan a design for the colored layers you will use, from bottom to top. Use a much larger soap mold to accommodate the many soap layers, or divide your recipe in half or thirds for each color of soap.

**2.** Using the Soap Esentials Bar II formula (or a similarly saturated formula), prepare the bottom layer of soap at your preferred soapmaking temperature. For a quick setup, it is critical that the soap is stirred *just* until definite trailings can be left on the surface. Quickly and thoroughly add desired scent; then pour into soapmaking mold. Place the mold on a thick comforter or blanket, cover with a tight-fitting top, and wrap with the comforter for good warm insulation.

**3.** Continue preparing and adding layers to the soap tray (waiting at least 1½ hours between layers, checking first for sufficient resistance), rewrapping the tray each time, until your final layer has undergone its full

**USING FRAGRANCE OILS**

The more reactive fragrance oils thicken the soap and set it too quickly when added at a full trace (pure essential oils are much more accommodating). If you are using fragrance oils, add at a very light trace. This process will still produce soap that hardens quickly enough for a rapid succession of layers, and the thinner consistency of the soap mixture makes perfectly level layers.

insulation period. Though the bottom layers can tolerate a few days enclosed in insulation, it is best to allow a more normal insulation period for each layer; once the final layer has been poured, allow the entire mass of soap to rest undisturbed under wrap for a full twelve to eighteen hours.

**4.** Trim and cure the bars as usual.

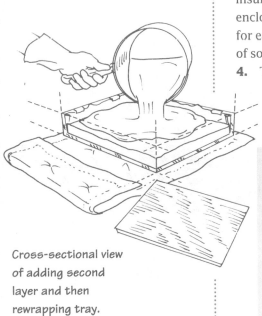

Cross-sectional view of adding second layer and then rewrapping tray.

### HOW LONG A WAIT BETWEEN LAYERS?

Some soapmakers wait a day between layers, but a formula with the proper balance of saturated and unsaturated fats and oils that has been stirred to a *full* trace (until you see definite trailings) produces a soap that hardens in time to accommodate a new layer 1½ to 2 hours after it is poured into the mold. The goal is to produce a soap that is hard enough to accept a new layer without buckling under the weight and blending colors.

Some soapmaking books recommend pouring new layers every twenty-four hours, but I try to avoid leaving any of the layers under wraps for longer than twenty-four hours. I like to get all of my layers poured as quickly as possible, with the final layer receiving at least twelve hours of insulation. Since my Soap Essentials Bar II formula (see pages 18–23) tolerates a new layer after just 1½ to 3 hours (with no bleeding!) when stirred to a *full* trace, I can add up to four layers of soap, without insulating the first layer for more than a total of twenty-four hours.

Layers can be spaced an hour and a half apart when the soap formula is sufficiently saturated and when the soap is stirred to a full trace. Trailings must remain on the surface of the soap instead of disappearing back into the mass for a soap mixture that sets up within an hour and a half. This well-traced soap is prone to thicken too quickly if the soapmaker does not act quickly while scenting and pouring the soap. Do not wait *past* the point of a full trace; add the scent just when the soap retains its first set of trailings.

## COBBLESTONE SOAP

Cobblestone soap is a beautiful way to recycle soap trimmings, scraps, and extra bars. It uses both finely shredded soap and irregular chunks of soap.

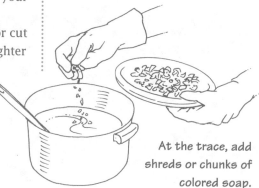

### Making Cobblestone Soap

**1.** Prepare and proceed to make your choice of soap formula as your base soap. I use a white base for the most striking contrast.

**2.** At the trace, incorporate 2 cups (500 ml) of long soap shreds or cut chunks of bar soap for every 5 pounds (2.3 kg) soap. Though lighter shreds can be added at a light or a full trace, heavier chunks of soap will sink to the bottom of thinly traced soap; they require a full trace for better suspension.

**3.** Complete the selected formula according to individual directions.

*At the trace, add shreds or chunks of colored soap.*

### TIPS FOR MAKING COBBLESTONE SOAP

◆ Use multicolored soap shreds and pieces for a more striking appearance.

◆ When using larger soap chunks, be sure to use soap that is not too hard; older soap is difficult to slice into chunks, and also more difficult to slice through when you are cutting and trimming the final bars.

◆ Cut the colorful soap into different-shaped chunks for an interesting effect.

◆ Add larger soap pieces once your base soap has reached a full trace. Thinly traced soap will not hold them in suspension.

◆ If scent is desired, add just before the soap pieces. If the pieces are scented, consider letting these alone scent the entire new batch lightly.

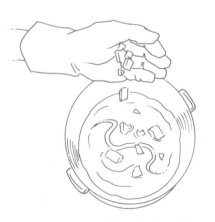

## STAINED-GLASS SOAP

We all have our favorite soaps, and this is one of mine. Stained-Glass Soap is closely related to Cobblestone Soap, but the contrasting chunks of color are pieces of transparent soap instead of opaque soap. The effect of irregular geometric shapes of transparent color on a white background is reminiscent of stained-glass windows on a sunny day.

I could visualize Stained-Glass Soap bars even before I had finalized my transparent formula. These beauties were the reward I looked forward to through weeks of trial and error. By the time the formula was right, I had accumulated lots of colored bars from my many experimental batches — all of the colors I needed for the finale. Since transparency is dependent upon a quick cool-down, I wondered if the small transparent pieces would become opaque when heated and cooled slowly within the new warm batch. They didn't. The colorful, transparent shapes appear to have the sun shining through them. Though I had imagined these bars for a while, the actual unveiling was nothing short of amazing.

### Making Stained-Glass Soap

**1.** This soap is fairly simple to make. For the most striking effect, gather as many colors of transparent soap as possible (preferably made within the last eight to twelve weeks, for easier cutting of the final bars); cut the transparent bars into pieces of irregular shape and size. Toss the pieces in a bowl to mix up the colors, and set the bowl aside.

**2.** Prepare a batch of basic white soap using a formula such as the Soap Essentials Bar II on pages 18–23 that hardens within eighteen to twenty-four hours. The key to success is waiting for a full trace; do not add the scent and the transparent pieces until some of the soap mixture drizzled from your spatula onto the surface remains there and holds its shape. The thin trace that works well for most plain batches would not hold the many chunks of transparent soap in suspension; they would all sink to the bottom of the mold. But a thicker emulsion keeps the pieces evenly dispersed as the soap hardens. Any scent should be added quickly just before the transparent pieces.

Once the soap has reached a full trace, add the transparent chunks.

**3.** Swiftly pour the soap into molds to avoid seizing.

**4.** Allow the soap an eighteen- to twenty-four-hour insulation period.

**5.** Cut the mass into bars and air-dry for three weeks.

## IMPRINTED SOAP

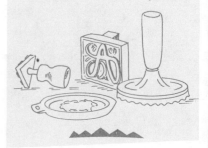

Milled animal- or vegetable-based soap (see chapter 9, pages 199–200) is easy to imprint, since certain synthetic chemicals make the soap rock hard and glossy, with all surfaces residue-free. Cold-process soap can be imprinted as well, but the results should not be compared to the crystal-clear impressions of its milled counterpart.

The best imprints are achieved by the cold-process soapmaker when beef or sheep tallow is included in the soapmaking formula. Only a rock-hard soap can be released from the stamp with a perfect impression of the pattern left behind. But all-vegetable soaps can be imprinted when formulas contain a high percentage of saturated fats such as palm oil, coconut oil, or palm kernel oil, or when a few ounces of beeswax or cocoa butter are added. Many formulas that contain high percentages of unsaturated oils can be imprinted after a few days of hardening, though the edges of the pattern may never be perfectly clean. Accept softer lines in place of perfectly defined ones and be patient with the process.

### Making Imprinted Soaps

Most of the soap formulas in this book can accept an imprint a day or two after the insulation period.

**1.** Prepare soap formula. Cut the soap into bars soon, if not immediately, after the insulation period.

**2.** Once all of the sides of each bar are hard and give way only to very firm pressure, the soap is ready for an impression. Test a small corner of a bar before proceeding. Once the stamp can be released cleanly, without taking some sticky soap with it, your soap is ready to be imprinted.

As soon as the sides of the bar are hard, it can be imprinted.

---

**TOOLS FOR CREATING AN IMPRINT**

A variety of utensils can be used for imprinting, including custom-made dies manufactured specifically for soapmaking, and stamps and presses borrowed from other crafts. The following tools are among the most accessible:

◆ Ceramic cookie stamps

◆ Metal stamps used on leather (I have a set of the letters of the alphabet, as well as other pretty patterns.)

◆ Hand-carved pieces of hardwood attached to a makeshift handle for easier stamping

## SOAP IN THE ROUND

Soapmakers eye all objects as potential soap molds. Like a photographer who cannot look at a scene without thinking about its possibilities as a photograph, the soapmaker is always on the lookout.

I still prefer rectangular chunks of soap. After all these years, I haven't tired of them. But some people like to make round, flat-bottomed bars using cylindrical molds of PVC (polyvinyl chloride) pipe. One end of the pipe is sealed before the soap is poured in; then the top end is sealed. The first person to think of this was clearly one of those soapmaking scouts I described above, for whom a quick trip to the hardware store presents a cornucopia of possibilities.

Soap in the Round is not for the soapmaker who expects today's batch to be the same as yesterday's and has no patience for stubborn batches that resist removal from the pipes. This technique is for the soapmaker who is willing to roll with the punches and accept the uncertainties of a makeshift attempt.

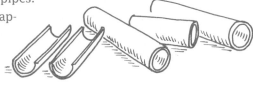

**Have PVC piping cut into 1- or 2-foot lengths.**

### Supplies/Mold Preparation

Begin by asking your local home center to cut the 10-foot (3-m) lengths of PVC pipe into convenient 1- or 2-foot (.3- or .6-m) lengths (approximately one pound of soap per one foot length of piping). If you are a soapmaker who is particularly frustrated by the occasional temperamental batch that may stick to the mold, ask about having the cut lengths of piping sliced vertically down the middle with a hacksaw. These halves can be temporarily sealed together until the soap is hard, at which point you remove the seal to easily pull the pipe halves away from the soap. There are several methods for sealing the ends of the pipe.

**Plastic wrap.** Seal the ends of the pipe with microwave-strength plastic wrap, double- or triple-folded for added resistance. Use heavy-duty rubber bands to hug the plastic wrap to the pipe and prevent leakage.

**Rubber bottom.** Some people seal the pipe's bottom end by placing the pipe on top of a sink plug or any other makeshift rubber or heavy-duty plastic piece that can be held to the pipe using candle mold seal (or another suitable clay).

**Wax.** Another option is using melted wax to plug the bottom of the pipe. Melt paraffin wax and pour it into a flat container to a height of ½ inch (1.27 cm). Set the pipe into the wax on its end and leave it until the wax hardens, at which time you can cut the pipe from the remainder of the wax. These leftover wax chunks can be used days later to push the sufficiently hardened soap out the other end of the pipe.

For multiple molds, melt a pound of wax in a baking pan set in a low-temperature oven. (Watch carefully to avoid overheating!) Once the wax has melted, take the pan from the oven and arrange the PVC pipes in the pan, with their open ends sunk into the molten wax. Let the wax harden at room temperature before adding the soap mixture. Cover the tops of the pipes as usual; the entire set of pipes should be set into a box and covered well with blankets during the insulation period. When the soap has hardened sufficiently you can break each pipe from the block, trim it a bit, and then use the wax plug to push the cylinder of soap from the PVC piping.

**Candle mold sealer.** If you are using pipes that have been sliced in half vertically, candle mold sealer does a nice job of sealing the seam after the two halves have been snugly reattached. This sealant also fills in any other gaps formed when rubber or other makeshift bottoms are attached to whole pieces of piping. To prepare the piping for filling, arrange the two halves as they were originally, and seal the seam with candle mold seal. Be sure to unroll the mold seal down the entire length of piping, stretching and pressing the edges firmly onto the piping for a tight seal. I have heard that modeling clay can be used, but I know from my candlemaking that the strongest mold seals are the most reliable. Three or four wrappings of heavy-duty duct tape around the patched piping hold the two halves together snugly and insulates the soap nicely. The ends should be prepared as described above.

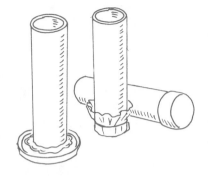

Three ways of sealing the bottom end of PVC pipe (r to l): wax, plastic wrap, and rubber bottom.

**CAUTION**

When melting wax in the oven, watch it carefully to avoid fire.

If you're using split PVC piping, seal the halves with candle mold sealer and wrap with duct tape before sealing the bottom.

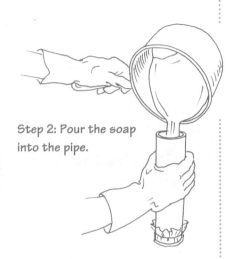

Step 2: Pour the soap into the pipe.

## Making Soap in the Round

**1.** Once the mold ends and sides are prepared according to any of the methods discussed under "Supplies/Mold Preparation," set them in a cardboard box or a cooler fitted with a blanket. Weave another blanket among the pipes to steady them.

**2.** Prepare the soap as usual and pour the traced soap mixture into the pipes, leaving a ½-inch (1.27-cm) gap between the top surface of the soap and the seal.

**3.** Seal the tops of the pipes accordingly; then use the other ends of the blankets to enclose the pipes snugly.

**4.** Close the cooler or the box and allow the soap to remain insulated for eighteen hours.

**5.** Remove the pipes and the top seal. When the soap appears sufficiently hard, remove the soap from the pipes (read the following section, "Unmolding Soap in the Round"), slice into rounds, and allow a three-week air-dry cure period.

### A NOTE ON INVENTIVE MOLDS

Molds of any size and shape can be perfectly custom-made by manufacturers, but makeshift alternatives provide a greater odyssey. With a little creativity and innovation, you can adapt a wide variety of materials to come close enough to replicating designs achieved with expensive molds. But be realistic and expect some fussing and fudging, while appreciating the little dents and bruises as signs of the human touch.

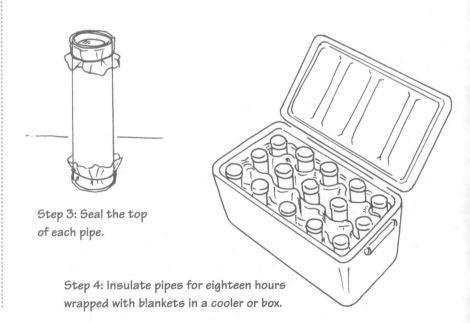

Step 3: Seal the top of each pipe.

Step 4: Insulate pipes for eighteen hours wrapped with blankets in a cooler or box.

## Unmolding Soap in the Round

**From Whole Pipes.** After the ease of peeling chunks of soap from heavy-duty waxed paper, you'll find coaxing soap from a plastic container to be a test of patience. Some highly saturated formulas produce a soap that releases more easily from the plastic walls. But more unsaturated formulas, or those that contain sticky nutrients such as honey, lanolin, or shea butter, are stubborn and resist movement.

Soap can only be unmolded successfully if it is sufficiently hard — much harder than soap molded in waxed paper needs to be before cutting and trimming. Some soapmakers grease the sides of the piping with vegetable shortening, vegetable sprays, or petroleum jelly, and push the hardened soap out using a round, flat-bottomed utensil. Attach a wooden dowel of some sort to a thick, round piece of plastic, wood, or any other hard, resistant material cut only a fraction smaller than the diameter of the piping. With a good, solid push, this plunger-type tool should push the soap through the piping after you break the seal.

A homemade plunger-type tool (using a wooden dowel attached to a round piece of wood) is useful for pushing soap from the piping.

### SELECTING A SOAP FORMULA

Most of your favorite soapmaking formulas can be used for making Soap in the Round, but if you are molding it in a whole pipe, I recommend a formula with a high percentage of saturated fats and oils. A soap that hardens quickly and resists impressions withstands the release process better than a softer, stickier soap. An ounce or two (25–50 g) of cocoa butter or beeswax is helpful. If you don't mind relying upon the freezer, you can use almost any soapmaking formula. I only use the freezer for transparent soap, and I do not like greasing molds with petroleum jelly, silicone spray, or vegetable shortening or sprays. Therefore, my soap itself must cooperate with the wax plunger toward its release from the mold.

If, however, you are molding in vertically split pipes from which soap is easily removed, you need not feel limited to using the more saturated formulas. Use any recipe of choice.

Still, soap and plastic cling to one another, and some batches are not helped even by greasing the surfaces. So some soapmakers skip the greasing step and rely upon the freezer to contract the soap away from the piping or — in the case of the most stubborn batches — to harden the soap enough to withstand a firmer push (see chapter 9, page 185). Once the soap has set for a day or so, and is sufficiently hard for unmolding, place the pipes in the freezer for about an hour. At this point, the block can usually be knocked out of the mold and left to cure at room temperature. If it can't, let the cold mold sit for around fifteen minutes or so, until condensation settles on the soap, then push the slippery soap from the mold. Also try rubbing a warm, damp towel that has been soaked in hot water and squeezed dry up and down and around the length of the piping.

**From Vertically Split Pipes.** When the soap has hardened sufficiently, these molds allow for easy removal. Simply unwrap the tape, strip off the mold seal (save it for next time), and lift off one of the halves of piping, then the other.

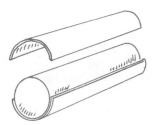

Removing soap from vertically split pipes is easy once you've unwrapped the duct tape and stripped off the seal.

## BURIED TREASURES

One night, after my mom brought us Chinese take-out food for dinner, complete with fortune cookies, I got the idea of tucking a message or trinket deep inside a bar of soap. I prefer messages to trinkets, and since I prefer personal notes to generic predictions, I've replaced warnings and promises with more intimate notes. A special label should accompany the finished bar of soap, notifying the recipient that a buried treasure waits within.

### Making Buried Treasures Soap

**1. Establish a grid.** The purpose of the grid is to ensure that you bury the treasure in the middle of the bars where you won't cut into it when you later slice the bars. To prepare a grid, use a simple piece of quilting plastic, or even tagboard or cardboard, the same size as your mold or tray. Draw a grid of the desired bar sizes (my bars are 5.8 cm x 7.6 cm) with lines ½ inch (1.27 cm) thick. Cut out the boxes between the lines.

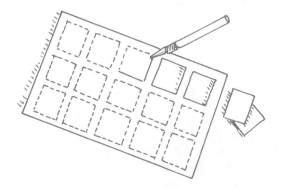

Make a grid from quilting template plastic or cardboard to fit your mold. Cut out the bar squares (step 1).

**2. Prepare the treasures.** Write little notes or find some trinkets you'd like to tuck inside of your soaps. Seal each note carefully in a tiny, heavy-duty plastic Zip-Loc bag (the kind that jewelers use for rings and earrings). Double-check each seal or the message will reach no one. Set the treasures aside until your soap is ready.

**3. Bury the treasures.** Prepare your favorite soap formula as usual. Most soap formulas allow you to bury the treasure without a problem. The key to success, once again, is pouring the soap after it reaches a fuller trace — not thick like pudding, but thick enough to hold a drizzled swirl of soap mixture on the surface. The emulsion must be stable enough to hold the package in suspension. Just after pouring the soap, lay the grid over the tray and use a small, nonpointed utensil such as a Popsicle stick to poke each treasure to the approximate center of each bar.

**4. Remove the grid.** Cover the tray and allow the soap its insulation period.

Bury a treasure in the center of each bar, poking it beneath the surface (step 3).

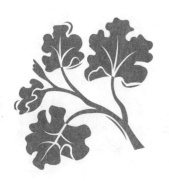

# CHAPTER 3
## Making Transparent Soaps

Though I had experimented with making transparent soaps a few years ago, I eventually abandoned the project because the best of them still seemed inferior to the opaque cold-process soaps I'd come to love. The transparent formulas incorporated alcohol, a drying ingredient, and they were produced at very high soapmaking temperatures, probably destroying some of the nutritive value of the vegetable oils. They were dangerous to produce, and because the formulas contained less soap and more liquid than opaque soap, they dissolved more quickly and affected the skin less beneficially.

But as I dispelled a few of my concerns and found ways around others, I wound my way back to these gems. I learned that I could use ethanol, a natural grain alcohol, and that most of it evaporates quickly from the soap. I learned that any transparent formula can be improved by including vegetable oils and nutrients. I learned that a carefully designed formula can produce longer-lasting soap, and that though opaque vegetable soap is usually finer, transparent bars can be made mild and pure and beneficial. The clincher involved no science at all, but rather an evolving sense that not all products have to be functional; some may be only aesthetic. These soaps are beautiful and gentle, and rather than ignore them because they offer less than the richest soap, I instead chose to explore their potential.

I have reworked a few turn-of-the-century transparent formulas, substituting vegetable-based materials for tallow and synthetics, and adjusting the ratios to accommodate a home-processing method. This method is very different from the industrial process that produces transparent soap in enclosed vessels.

## THE STORY OF TRANSPARENT SOAP

Transparent soap has become synonymous with glycerin soap, and yet there is a distinction to be made. Under the umbrella of "glycerin soap" fall many soaps, including transparent. The cold-process opaque soaps described in Chapter 1 and in *The Natural Soap Book* are glycerin soaps, because they retain the glycerin produced during saponification. Some soap manufacturers, who make soap using fatty acids that have been split from the glycerol portion of the triglyceride, add glycerin — usually a synthetic glycerin — to their soap formulas and call the results glycerin soaps. And some companies label their translucent and transparent soaps as glycerin soaps because they contain various polyols (kinds of alcohols), one of which is often glycerin.

I distinguish between glycerin/opaque soap, translucent soap, and transparent soap. I define *glycerin soap* as cold-process opaque soap that retains the natural glycerin produced during the soapmaking process. This opaque soap diffuses light and does not allow any to pass through. *Translucent soap* is neither opaque nor transparent; it scatters some light, but allows a little to pass through, as a lampshade does. A deep haze keeps translucent soap from being see-through, though it is clearer than opaque soap. *Transparent soap* is the clearest of all. It transmits light with little scattering, so some objects beyond are visible. A person with good vision should be able to see large objects through a transparent bar of soap. Within the industry, a generally accepted standard defines transparency: The 14-point print on a business card should be legible through a ¼-inch (.6-cm) slice of transparent soap. The bar as a whole will be light and glossy and free of obstruction, though not as perfectly clear as a slice of the bar.

Transparent soap is clear enough to read medium-sized type through.

## Beginnings

Transparent soap was first developed in Great Britain in the late 1700s, known then and now as Pears transparent soap. Though these bars are rare among cold-process soapmakers, they've been produced industrially for a long time, with varying degrees of popularity. On the whole, transparent soap has never been as popular as other soaps, because it does not last as long and is typically more expensive. Still, because people think of it as "natural," it is revived with other natural products during each back-to-basics movement.

## Keys to Production

Opaque cold-process soap consists of tightly enmeshed fibers that form during a slow cure at warm temperatures. The trick in producing transparent soap is to avoid the formation of these fibers. Polyglycols — alcohol, sugar, and vegetable glycerin — are added to saponified soap to dilute, clear, and brighten the soap. Castor oil, one of the soapmaking oils, also produces transparency. The raw materials used, such as fats, oils, colorants, and essential or fragrance oils, must have as little color as possible, to keep the soap clear and glossy. Cooling the finished mixture quickly prevents the formation of the fibrous crystals that block the passage of light. Transparency requires limited crystal growth; the soap crystals must be smaller than the wavelengths of light.

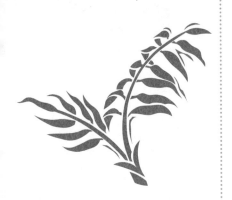

Opaque soap can be made transparent when mixed with alcohols under certain conditions. These alcohols are referred to as polyols, and include a variety of substances, such as glycerin, ethyl alcohol, and sugars. A polyol, known formally as a polyhydric alcohol, is an alcohol that contains three or more hydroxyl groups. A hydroxyl group — symbolized by OH — is a combination of one atom of hydrogen bound chemically to one atom of oxygen. Those polyols with only three OH groups (trihydric) are glycerols.

A well-designed transparent formula is critical, with careful attention paid to two different ratios: that of soap (the saponified product from the reaction of fats and oils and lye) to polyols, and that of one polyol to another. The perfect balance produces a reliable transparency. Too much glycerin or sugar syrup makes a sticky, soft soap that sweats. Too much alcohol makes a harsh soap with a strong alcohol odor. Too much soap in proportion to the rest of the formula makes an opaque bar instead of a transparent one. Too much liquid prevents the mixture from hardening. Transparent formulas are not forgiving; there is little to no margin for error.

Because I choose to avoid synthetic intrusion, my soap is aesthetically inferior to its synthetic counterpart. Though the soap is perfectly transparent, I have been unable to create a natural transparent soap that does not experience some shrinkage due to the evaporation of the polyols used for transparency. As the alcohol required for transparency evaporates, the bars shrink. Within industry, a variety of synthetics — including triethanolamine — produce transparency without affecting the bar's size or appearance. I'd rather make the purest bar possible, polish it once it has cured, and accept some shrinkage.

## ETHANOL (ETHYL ALCOHOL) AND THE HOME SOAPMAKING PROCESS

Transparent soap is made using a variety of methods and materials. To achieve transparency, one or more polyols must be incorporated into the soapmaking formula, but a few combinations are possible. The synthetic alcohols such as triethanolamine are selected by industry not only for better aesthetics, but also because they are easy to use and have higher flash points. Ethyl alcohol has a very low flash point and is highly combustible, so a soapmaker must be especially careful when using it. In an effort to produce a nonsynthetic product, I have chosen to use a grain alcohol — natural ethanol — but I make this transparent soap in very small batches to keep the risks to a minimum.

Alcohol has always been a critical ingredient for transparency, but with its low flash point, it is dangerous to expose alcohol to the combination of heat and oxygen. Industry avoids alcohol entirely by substituting synthetic materials or it minimizes the risk by producing the soap in an enclosed system, pumping the alcohol and the other ingredients into the soapmaking vessel without any exposure to air. *Do not increase your batches to mass-production sizes without first researching the enclosed vessels needed to produce large quantities of soap made with alcohol.*

I would rather not make a soap than uses synthetic polyols, so I have chosen to experiment with alcohol. Of course, fire is the most significant

**Flash point**

The lowest temperature at which the vapors of a volatile material, like ethanol, ignite in the presence of a spark.

risk of all, far outweighing the risk of synthetic intrusion. But by making very small batches and by self enforcing safety standards, I've been able to make transparent soap in my home. Still, no level of comfort should ever creep into the process. Be intensely alert when making each and every batch of transparent soap with alcohol, and do not let yourself become even one iota complacent.

Be sure to use minimal water, so there will be less need for you to cook down the mixture. Alcohol should not be exposed to heat for long. Aside from the risk of fire, too much alcohol is lost to evaporation when a soap mixture is overheated; the alcohol is needed to prevent the formation of large crystals.

## What is Ethanol?

When most of us think of alcohol, we think of ethanol — the alcohol in alcoholic beverages, such as beer, wine, and brandy. But *alcohol* is a chemical term. It is a chain of carbon and hydrogen atoms with one or more hydroxyl (OH) groups attached to it. Ethanol is one kind of alcohol; it has only one hydroxyl group. Glycols are alcohols with two hydroxyl groups; and glycerin is an alcohol with three hydroxyl groups. Alcohols have an unequal distribution of charges in the C–O–H part of their structure, and this arrangement is responsible for many of their physical and chemical properties.

Ethanol, also known as ethyl alcohol, and symbolized by $C_2H_5OH$, is a clear, colorless, flammable alcohol. All beverage ethanol is made by fermenting sugar or starch, a natural process that occurs when living cells are broken down in the absence of oxygen. A yeast enzyme, zymase, converts the simple sugars within potatoes, corn, or other cereals into ethanol and carbon dioxide. The chemical equation is as follows:

$$C_6H_{12}O_6 \longrightarrow 2C_2H_5OH + 2CO_2$$

| simple sugars | ferment naturally to produce | ethanol | and | carbon dioxide |

It can also be produced synthetically, but this form is not recommended for use within the formulas that follow. This alcohol is antiseptic, antibacterial, and cooling, but can also be drying to hair and skin.

Ethanol is around 95 percent pure, with approximately 5 percent water. The concentration of an ethyl alcohol is expressed as proof, which is simply twice the volume percent of ethyl alcohol. For example, 190-proof ethanol is 95 percent ethyl alcohol, and 100-proof whiskey is 50 percent ethyl alcohol. The purchase of ethyl alcohol for drinking or production purposes is closely monitored by the federal government. Soapmakers and distillers alike must follow strict guidelines. I have decided not to produce transparent soap on a large scale, so I purchase my grain alcohol from the liquor store and pay a high tax for the convenience.

## DENATURED ALCOHOL

A much less expensive alcohol to use in manufacturing transparent soap is denatured alcohol. Ethanol is taxed because it is used to manufacture alcoholic beverages. But a denatured alcohol is a nontaxable item because it has been deliberately poisoned to make it undrinkable. Toxic, malodorous chemicals, such as denatonium benzoate, are added to the ethanol to ensure that the end user will certainly not drink it, but instead use it to produce soap, pesticides, synthetic rubber, detergents, or lubricants. Denatured alcohol is the inexpensive choice of many manufacturers, but it is not an acceptable skin-care substitute for pure ethanol. The term *SD alcohol* reveals that the alcohol was "specially denatured." Avoid these denatured alcohols and synthetically prepared ethanol.

There are, however, denatured alcohols that can be used by natural-cosmetic companies. These contain pure essential oils that soapmakers routinely include in their soap formulas. To 100 gallons (378.5 liters) of ethanol, 10 pounds (4.54 kg) of one or more designated essential oils are added to make the ethanol dangerous to consume. This denatured version of ethanol does not undergo a synthetic process and does not contain synthetic materials. It is a less expensive alternative to ethanol for those soapmakers who produce enough transparent soap

### PURCHASING ETHANOL IN QUANTITY

Those who want to purchase alcohol from chemical supply companies must register with the Federal Bureau of Alcohol, Tobacco, and Firearms and purchase an alcohol permit. Ethanol, because it is a beverage alcohol, cannot be purchased tax-free, even with an alcohol permit. But denatured alcohol — ethanol that has been altered with materials that make it unfit to drink — can be purchased inexpensively and tax-free. The requirements are many and ongoing, but the tax savings is substantial.

to justify the yearly cost of an alcohol permit, as well as the hassle of complying with regulations and submitting records. Those who choose ethanol over any of the denatured alcohols available must pay the tax, though they can file for a drawback, which is a refund of approximately 90 percent. Once the ethanol has been purchased and used in production, a percentage of the portion used is credited by the government.

## SAFETY PRECAUTIONS

With its very low vapor pressure and flash point, ethanol must be treated with the utmost care and caution. I have dealt with it carefully while experimenting and have never experienced a problem. Of course, I don't know how close I've come to disaster.

Using ethanol at high temperatures can be compared to setting a match to the brandy in crêpes suzettes for a flaming presentation at the table. The analogy is dangerously inaccurate, however. A flaming dessert is much safer than a heated transparent soap mixture. There is far less alcohol in the dessert, and the alcohol is lower proof.

There's no way around it. At this point in time, the soapmaker has four options: to make soap using synthetic polyols with higher flash points (these, too, are extremely flammable, though their flash points are higher than ethanol's); to design a room with hermetically sealed ignition sources such as light fixtures and switches and to design a closed system in which the ethanol has no contact with oxygen; to make very small batches of transparent soap using the transparent formulas designed for hobbyists while exercising great caution; or to choose to make opaque bars, instead of the transparent ones.

Most of us know not to light a match near alcohol, the way we would not light a match near the gas pumps at a gas station. But a spark is not the only way to start a fire around ethanol. The vapor itself is extremely flammable, so it is important to prevent the congregation of fumes in one small area. The vapor is lighter than air, so a vapor pool will rise to the top of a building. The problem lies less with the gently simmering materials in the soapmaking pan, and more with the alcoholic vapor. The soap

**Vapor pressure**

The amount of pressure exerted by a substance in its gaseous state (when the substance is in equilibrium with its solid and liquid state).

mixture will not spontaneously ignite; ignition requires a source, in the form of heavily concentrated fumes.

In the worst-case scenario, a large vapor pool forms near an ignition source and bursts into flame. Industry protects against such an occurrence by following rigorous safety precautions. Factories are equipped with fire walls, enclosed fixtures, and sprinkler systems. The large quantities of ethanol used industrially produce huge vapor pools that could ignite with just the flip of a switch.

Since I am not confident that I can prevent disaster in a home setting, I do not make large batches that incorporate large quantities of ethanol. Instead, I make only a dozen transparent bars at a time, using not much more alcohol than is used in the flaming dessert. By opening windows or by using a large enough room, the small amount of vapor produced is dispersed across an adequate area. This way, the vapors do not accumulate in one spot; they spread out and minimize the risk. Of course, never light a match near the soap mixture.

No doubt some of you think I'm overreacting. I'm not.

## MAKING TRANSPARENT SOAP

To make a transparent soap, a mixture is first made using the opaque soap process, but with high temperatures and without superfatting the formula. Castor oil, one of the soapmaking oils, contributes to transparency. It is important for transparency that no excess fats and oils are left in the final bars, so this soap mixture must be fully saponified. After saponification, a combination of polyols is added for transparency, including vegetable glycerin, a sugar syrup (made from dissolving sugar in boiling water), and ethanol, the alcohol.

Transparent soap carefully balances the ratio of soap to polyols. Too high a percentage of soap to the polyol portion will make an opaque soap. Too low a percentage will make sticky, mushy soap. After much experimentation, I settled on 55 percent soap and 45 percent polyols.

Different transparent formulas use different soapmaking processes. Some add the alcohol to the lye solution from the start (not my recommendation); some include rosin, a resin obtained from pine trees or pine

**SAFETY CHECKLIST**

❏ Good ventilation enabling the continuous exchange of fresh air for inside air.
❏ No sparks nearby (no smoking; do not light a match). Use an electric stove only.
❏ Fire extinguisher nearby.
❏ Any overhead lighting directly above the soapmaking pan is turned off.

stumps; some use glycerin, but not the sugar syrup or the alcohol, while others choose one, two, or all three of these polyols; and some allow the soap to rest for a couple of hours before adding the polyols. I experimented with many of the possibilities before settling on the formula included here.

## Equipment

◆ Electric stove
◆ Plastic rectangular mold (Rubbermaid or Tupperware quality, approximately 8" x 5" x 2" [20 x 12.7 x 5 cm]), or plastic molds of choice
◆ Three small glass measuring cups with pouring spouts
◆ Three small containers to hold the vegetable glycerin, sodium hydroxide, and sugar
◆ Freestanding mixer with splash-guard (optional)
◆ 3-quart (3-l) heavy-duty stainless steel or enamel saucepan (never aluminum or cast iron), called "the soapmaking pan"
◆ Small saucepan in which to melt the coconut oil and palm oil
◆ 12-cup (3-l) heat-proof glass bowl with pouring lip
◆ One good-quality thermometer (0–220°F [18–104°C]); the quick-read type is best
◆ Rubber spatula

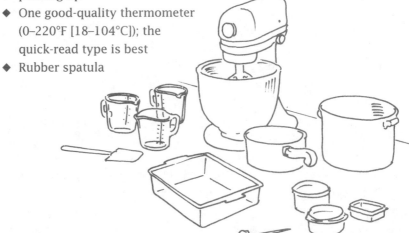

## "SUN ON GLASS" TRANSPARENT SOAP
### Makes nine 3-ounce (85-g) bars

Ｍy favorite use of transparent soap is Stained-Glass Soap (see page 70), an opaque white soap dotted with colored transparent pieces. Most of my batches of this soap are saved for the day when I have six to ten colors to incorporate into that delightful creation.

In this formula, the soap portion weighs 618 grams (55 percent) and the polyol portion weighs 506.4 grams (45 percent). Of the polyol portion only, alcohol constitutes 46 percent, sugar syrup constitutes 35.4 percent, and glycerin constitutes 18.6 percent. Small batches are more accurately measured in metric units.

### Polyol Mixture
94.2 grams (3.3 ounces) vegetable glycerin
101.4 grams (3.5 ounces) quick-dissolving sugar
232.8 grams (8.1 ounces) ethanol (Everclear brand)
78 grams (2.7 ounces) distilled water

### Fats and Oils
138 grams (4.8 ounces) coconut oil
138 grams (4.8 ounces) palm oil
117 grams (4 ounces) castor oil

### Lye Solution
72 grams (2.5 ounces) sodium hydroxide
153 grams (5.4 ounces) cold distilled water

3 teaspoons (15 ml) pure essential oil or fragrance, optional

**1.** First, review all of the safety precautions (see pages 84–85).
**2.** Using a gram scale, measure out the vegetable glycerin and the sugar into two separate containers and set aside.
**3.** Weigh the correct amount of ethanol into one of the glass measuring cups and cover tightly with plastic wrap.

### A FEW TRANSPARENT SCENT BLENDS
Use 3 teaspoons (15 ml) of any of the following essential or fragrance oil blends to scent one batch of the transparent soap formula.

**Blend A**
| | |
|---|---|
| Geranium | ¼ teaspoon (1.25 ml) |
| Cassia | ½ teaspoon (2.5 ml) |
| Lavender | ¾ teaspoon (3.75 ml) |
| Sandalwood | 1½ teaspoons (7.5 ml) |

**Blend B**
| | |
|---|---|
| Lavender | 1½ teaspoons (7.5 ml) |
| Thyme | ¾ teaspoon (3.75 ml) |
| Cumin | ¾ teaspoon (3.75 ml) |

**Blend C**
| | |
|---|---|
| Lavender | 1⅜ teaspoons (6.9 ml) |
| Spike lavender | ⅞ teaspoon (4.4 ml) |
| Geranium | ¼ teaspoon (1.25 ml) |
| Patchouli | ¼ teaspoon (1.25 ml) |
| Palmarosa | ¼ teaspoon (1.25 ml) |

**Blend D**
| | |
|---|---|
| Geranium | ⅜ teaspoon (1.9 ml) |
| Lemon | ⅜ teaspoon (1.9 ml) |
| Palmarosa | 2 teaspoons (10 ml) |
| Bergamot | ¼ teaspoon (1.25 ml) |

**4.** To make the sugar syrup, add the 78 grams of water to measuring cup containing sugar. Heat in the microwave for around thirty seconds on high until the water just comes to a boil. Remove the cup and dissolve the sugar by stirring very quickly. Seal the cup tightly with microwave plastic wrap or foil until you are ready to use it.

**5.** Set the small saucepan on the scale and add the correct weights of coconut, palm, and castor oils. Set aside.

**6.** Into the third small glass measuring cup, add the 153 grams of cold water. Into a small container, weigh out the sodium hydroxide. Thoroughly dissolve the sodium hydroxide in the water, stirring quickly. Set aside to cool to 120–130°F (49–54.4°C).

**7.** Heat the fats and oils at a medium-high setting until the coconut and palm oils have melted (no need to stir).

**8.** When the fats/oils and the lye solution both reach around 120–130°F (49–54.4°C), drizzle the lye solution into the fats/oils and stir very quickly (as quickly as possible when stirring by hand; when using an electric mixer with a splash-guard, set on speed 2 at first, then speed 3, and eventually even 4 as the soap becomes progressively thicker). Unlike opaque soap, this soap must thicken to the fullest trace, more like a light pudding. This tiny batch takes around fifteen minutes to saponify in the electric mixer.

**9.** When the soap is good and thick, use a spatula to scrape it into the 3-quart (3-l) soapmaking pan. Add the vegetable glycerin to the soap and stir gently over a medium-low setting (setting 3) of an electric stove until the soap reaches 130°F (54.4°C). **Remove the pan from the stove** and drizzle in the alcohol.

**10.** Place pan back on the stove at a medium-low setting, and with minimum intrusion do what I call "scrunching." Until the soap melts and combines with the alcohol, it will float above the alcohol in solid clumps. Do not stir this mixture, but scrunch it with a rubber spatula (gently mash and melt it into the solution). Continue until the soap mixture and the alcohol melt into a uniform blend, or until the mixture reaches 160°F (71°C). If the liquid reaches this temperature, remove the pan from the heat and scrunch the final few pieces of soap while off the stove.

To combine the soap and alcohol, scrunch gently with a spatula. Do not stir.

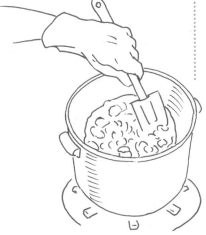

**11.** Reheat the sugar syrup for thirty seconds on the high setting in the microwave, to approximately 160°F (71°C). Set the soapmaking pan back on the burner and check to be sure the temperature is close to 160°F (71°C). If it has cooled somewhat, heat the soap mixture before adding the 160°F (71°C) sugar syrup. *Slowly* blend the sugar syrup and the soap mixture, using only three or four gentle strokes of the spatula. Do not stir, or the bubbles will affect the final soap.

**12.** When the soap mixture reaches 180°F (82°C) and a film begins to form on its surface, remove soap mixture from the heat. If any small pieces of soap remain, gently scrunch them into the solution. Work quickly, though gently. The goal is to pour soon after removing the soap from the heat. Ignore the small amount of foam that is soon strained from the soap.

**13.** Pour the soap mixture through a small-mesh strainer (the finest mesh you can find) into a heat-proof glass bowl. Pour slowly, leaving any film, foam, or solids behind in the pan. Gently stir in the essential oil, blending well. Using a clean strainer, strain the soap once more as it is poured into the plastic mold.

**14.** Immediately place the soap tray in the coldest part of the freezer for ¾–1 hour, or until the soap is hard through the center (gently press down on the center to test for resistance).

**15.** Pop the frozen soap out of the mold onto a cutting board (this is fun and easy compared to unmolding stubborn opaque vegetable soap from a plastic mold). Cut the soap into bars, and trim any film or stable lather off the top of each bar. Let the bars rest at room temperature for two weeks, allowing time for the excess alcohol and water to evaporate.

**16.** Using a lint-free cloth soaked in ethanol, polish the bars. Allow the soap to rest for two weeks to evaporate the excess alcohol and water; then use a lint-free towel soaked in ethanol to wipe any residual moisture from the bars.

Pour the final soap mixture through a fine-mesh strainer, and then strain again when pouring into the mold.

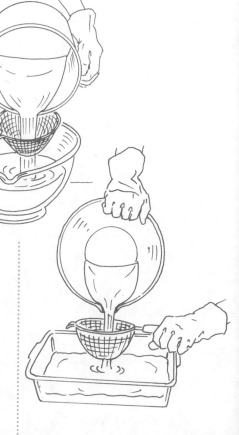

## Developing Your Own Variations

Once you understand how to achieve transparency, you can begin to design interesting variations of the basic formula. The ratio of soap to polyols and the ratio of one polyol to another must remain constant, but different fats and oils and nutrients can be substituted for those in "Sun on Glass" Transparent Soap. Choose substitutes that are equally clear, or the final soap will not be as transparent. Also, do not adjust the percentage of castor oil.

Of course, if you have a favorite nutrient, colorant, essential oil, or fatty oil that is somewhat cloudy, include it anyhow and accept the imperfect results in exchange for what may turn out to be your favorite soap. Here is one of my own variations.

Any time you substitute one fat or oil for another, be sure to rework the required amount of sodium hydroxide for a complete saponification. Never take a sodium hydroxide discount. *Fully* saponified soap contributes to transparency; excess oils cloud the final bars.

## STAINED-GLASS SOAP

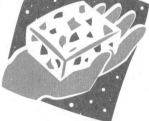

I like this soap even more than a whole transparent bar because the soap base is my favorite skin-care formula (opaque vegetable) and because the perfectly transparent colors against the white background are beautiful. See Chapter 2, page 70 for recipe.

# SILKY SEE-THROUGH SOAP

This soap is more emollient than a basic transparent bar with fats and oils chosen for their moisturizing qualities. The wheat germ oil contributes a yellow-orange color to the soap, so I often scent it with a sweet orange/citrus blend. The shea butter and the cocoa butter produce a silky lather.

**Polyol Mixture**
94.1 grams (3.3 ounces) vegetable glycerin
77.9 grams (2.7 ounces) distilled water
101.2 grams (3.5 ounces) quick-dissolving sugar
232.8 grams (8.1 ounces) ethanol (Everclear)

**Fats and Oils**
17.5 grams (.6 ounces) wheat germ oil
17.5 grams (.6 ounces) shea butter
70.1 grams (2.5 ounces) cocoa butter
35.1 grams (1.2 ounces) palm oil
140.2 grams (4.9 ounces) coconut oil
120.1 grams (4.2 ounces) castor oil

**Lye Solution**
156.4 grams (5.5 ounces) distilled water
61.4 grams (2.1 ounces) sodium hydroxide

3 teaspoons (15 ml) pure essential oil or fragrance oil, optional

Follow the instructions for "Sun on Glass" Transparent Soap on pages 87–89.

## SHIMMERS AND CURLS

Another fun soap to make using transparent soap is an opaque or transparent base bar covered with shredded homemade transparent soap. Commercial transparent soap is too hard and brittle to shred into soft flexible shreds, but my formula produces shiny, perfectly transparent shreds that form gel-like curly-Q's as they extrude through the hand-shredder.

These are beautiful guest bathroom bars. Once used, the transparent shreds are flattened, but until then, Shimmers and Curls are delightful. **To make:** Set aside fully cured bars of soap (transparent, opaque, or stained glass) for the base of Shimmers and Curls. Hand-shred two different colors of transparent soap and gently mix the two without squashing the pieces. Mound a handful of shreds on top of the wet transparent soap layer and gently press the shreds in place. Drizzle some melted transparent soap through the shreds to keep them in place.

## CREATING COLORFUL TRANSPARENCY

Color must be judiciously added to transparent soap. The inclusion of insoluble colors obstructs light and inhibits transparency. The best colorants are those that can be steeped in the lye solution before the lye is strained and added to the fats and oils, including madder root, brazilwood, and chlorophyll; and those that release their color in warm fats and oils, such as annatto seed and alkanet root. Less ideal, but still beautiful, are the ultramarines. As pigments, they impair transparency, but a good job of straining the powder before adding it to the soap controls the degree of obstruction. Be sure to strain the lye solution and the fats once the color has been released. The following colors can be added to the transparent formula on page 87. Or read chapter 5, "Using Natural Colorants," and experiment with other possibilities. Make a variety of colored batches for a spectacular display of Stained-Glass Soap (see chapter 2, page 70).

## A FEW COLOR SUGGESTIONS

| Color | Formula |
| --- | --- |
| Gray-lavender | 3 teaspoons (15 ml) alkanet root flakes into lye solution |
| Orange-red | ½ teaspoon (2 ml) ground madder root into lye solution |
| Brandy color | ¾ teaspoon (3 ml)  ground brazilwood into lye solution |
| Green | ½–3 teaspoons (2–15 ml) oil-soluble chlorophyll into warm oils (strain before use) |
| Bright yellow | 1–1½ tablespoons (15–22.5 ml) annatto seeds into warm oils (strain before use) or ¼ teaspoon (1 ml) powdered annatto dissolved into lye solution, or few drops oil-soluble annatto extract into oils or tracing soap |
| Purple (use less lavender) | 1½–2 grams ultramarine violet into lye solution (force ultramarine pigment through finest-mesh tea strainer) |
| Robin's-egg blue | 1½ grams ultramarine blue into lye solution (strained as described above for ultramarine violet) |

## THE SEARCH FOR A PERFECT TRANSPARENT SOAP

Recently, I received from soapmaker Catherine Failor the first draft of her book, *Transparent Soapmaking*. Catherine, an experienced soapmaker who specializes in transparent soap, keeps shrinkage to a minimum by using less alcohol in an innovative, homemade version of the enclosed system used by industrial soapmakers. Catherine's process is more involved than my short-cut, but the extra labor produces bars that perfectly retain their shape during the cure. Her higher ratio of soap to polyols creates a fuller skin-care offering. I have been thrilled with the perfect transparency and texture of my bars, and they make lovely gems for Stained-Glass Soap, but if you are looking for perfection, take the time to make Catherine's soap.

Catherine's writing is clear and concise, fun and fresh. With plenty of recipes and variations, and a thorough discussion of the process, Catherine has shared something unique in her new book. For more information, contact Rose City Press (see page 273 for address).

# TROUBLESHOOTING GUIDE TO TRANSPARENT SOAPS

| Problem | Possible Causes |
|---|---|
| Cloudiness | ◆ Added polyols before soap had fully saponified<br>◆ Not enough sodium hydroxide used (incomplete saponification — the free fats and oils cause the cloudiness)<br>◆ Cloudy fats and oils<br>◆ Mixture not cooled quickly enough |
| Opacity | ◆ Loss of alcohol due to evaporation<br>◆ Insufficient sugars or glycerin<br>◆ Insoluble materials in the colorant or scent<br>◆ Soapmaking temperatures too low<br>◆ Impurities in the raw materials |
| Softness | ◆ Too much water<br>◆ Not enough sodium hydroxide<br>◆ Not enough time allowed for saponification<br>◆ Too high a percentage of polyols to the percentage of soap |
| Alcoholic odor | ◆ Too much alcohol used |
| Slippery, hard feel to the soap | ◆ Too much alcohol used |
| Solid foam on top of final soap | ◆ Stable foam not scrunched during processing |
| Excessive shrinkage | ◆ Too much water and/or alcohol (evaporation) |
| Excessive sweating | ◆ Too much glycerin or sugar |

# CHAPTER 4
## An Overview of Soapmaking Oils

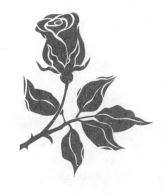

Many fats and oils are available to the soapmaker — some common and others obscure — all of which can produce soap. Neem oil and rosa mosqueta rose hip seed oil react with lye to make soap. So do olive oil, tallow, bacon grease, and vegetable shortening. Soapmakers are less limited by chemistry than they are by cost and availability.

Soapmakers are responsible for the recent availability of 35-pound pails of palm oil. In the past, palm oil was purchased almost exclusively by mass-producers, so there was little demand for quantities smaller than palettes and drums. A flood of soapmakers have recently rushed manufacturers and distributors into a whole new market, and we can now find 35-pound pails of sesame, hemp seed, and pumpkin seed oils.

I am grateful to have easy access to palm oil, so I do not complain that hemp seed oil is unaffordable as a majority oil or that it is nearly impossible to purchase palm kernel oil in less than drum quantities. Supply and demand determines availability, and until there is a demand for less-popular oils, cost stays high and availability is sporadic. Overall, availability has never been better for the small soapmaker than it is now. The large manufacturers and distributors often carry a wider range of fats and oils, though higher-priced, specialty companies offer the more unusual ingredients in smaller quantities. Buyer guides, like those listed in the appendix, list the larger suppliers of soapmaking ingredients. Bad news may follow when you phone for minimums, but one of the companies may be happy to share the names of customers who sell in smaller quantities. It's effort, but it usually works.

The essential nature of any soap is directly related to the oils and fats within. Only by understanding the benefits and limitations of each one can the soapmaker determine which combinations are effective and most feasible. The following descriptions are designed to help you create the best formulations.

## SOAP CHARACTERISTICS PRODUCED BY VARIOUS FATS AND OILS

| Fat/Oil | Hard Bar | Cleansing | Fluffy Lather | Stable Lather | Condi- tioning | Quick Trace |
|---|---|---|---|---|---|---|
| Almond (sweet) oil | | | | X | X | |
| Apricot kernel oil | | | | X | X | |
| Babassu oil | X | X | X | | | X |
| Borage oil | | | | X | X | |
| Calendula oil | | | | X | X | |
| Canola/Rapeseed oil | | | | X | X | |
| Castor oil | | | | X | X | X |
| Cocoa butter | X | | | X | X | X |
| Coconut oil | X | X | X | | | X |
| Corn oil | | | | X | X | |
| Cottonseed oil | | | | X | | |
| Evening primrose oil | | | | X | X | |
| Hazelnut oil | | | | X | X | |
| Hemp seed oil | | | | X | X | |
| Jojoba oil | | | | X | X | |
| Kukui nut oil | | | | X | X | |
| Lanolin | X | | | | X | X |
| Lard | X | | | X | X | X |
| Macadamia nut oil | | | | X | X | |
| Neem oil | | | | X | X | |
| Olive oil | | | | X | X | |
| Palm kernel oil | X | X | X | | | X |
| Palm oil | X | | | X | | X |
| Peanut oil | | | | X | X | |
| Safflower oil | | | | X | X | |
| Sesame oil | | | | X | X | |
| Shea butter | X | | | X | X | X |
| Soybean oil (veg. oil) | | | | X | X | |
| Soybean oil — hydrogenated (veg. shortening) | | | | X | X | |
| Sunflower oil | | | | X | X | |
| Tallow | X | | | X | X | X |
| Vegetable shortening | | | | X | X | |
| Wheat germ oil | | | | X | X | |

## A NOTE ON THIS CHART

This chart is narrowly drawn for the purpose of comparison. More generally, all fats and oils contribute some degree of each soap characteristic. For instance, beef tallow soap cleans, coconut oil soap conditions, and olive oil soap hardens, though other fats and oils clean, condition, and harden better (as indicated on this chart).

## AVOCADO OIL

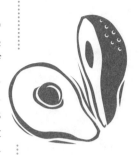

**Nature/Benefits:** Avocado oil is obtained from the pulp of the avocado pear and is one of the most active and effective ingredients used by the cosmetic industry. Because it has an extraordinarily high percentage of *unsaponifiables* (the portion of the oil which does not react to form soap, but rather retains its original makeup), avocado oil is highly therapeutic. It contains protein, amino acids, and relatively large amounts of vitamins A, D, and E, making this oil very much alive. These components are not only moisturizing, but also healing. They enable avocado oil to regenerate cells, soften body tissue, and heal scaly skin and scalp.

**Use in Soapmaking:** As with almond oil, avocado oil need not be the predominant oil in a soap formula for the benefits of its qualities to be enjoyed. Don't rely upon this oil for lather or hardness, but instead for its effective unsaponifiables. Splurge and use higher proportions of avocado oil in the base formula in soap for people with extremely sensitive skin.

## CALENDULA OIL

**Nature/Benefits:** Calendula, also known as pot marigold, is an herb whose blossoms yield calendula oil, known for its skincare properties. For therapeutic benefits, be sure to use only the pure oil extracted without solvents. Calendula oil's regenerative and anti-inflammatory properties are known to successfully heal a variety of types of skin damage. The oil promotes the healing of wounds, burns, and tissue, and softens and soothes dry, chapped skin.

**Use in Soapmaking:** To use calendula as a superfatting nutrient, add 1⅔ tablespoons for every 5 pounds of soap just before adding the essential oils. For a greater benefit, add 10 to 20 percent calendula oil (of the total fats and oils) to the other liquid oils at the start of the soapmaking process.

## CANOLA OIL

**Nature/Benefits:** Canola is a kind of rapeseed, a cultivar of *Brassica napus linnaeus,* and an ancient cross of two other genetically related species. It is a member of the mustard family, from which a variety of rapeseed oils are obtained. The canola cultivar produces seed with high oil and protein contents, and a low–erucic acid content. Most rapeseed plants produce high–erucic acid oils that are not approved as edible, and are only used within industry as lubricants, nylon components, and plastics components. Canola oil contains only 6 percent saturated fatty acids, making it lower in saturated fat than any other edible oil.

**Use in Soapmaking:**  Without saturated fatty acids, high–oleic acid canola oil can be slower to saponify. Still, in combination with other saturated fats and oils, it can replace a portion of more costly oils while contributing protein and moisturizing qualities. Due to its relatively low SAP value (see chapter 13, page 247), be especially careful to adjust the sodium hydroxide measurements when substituting it for most other oils.

### CASTOR OIL

**Nature/Benefits:**  The castor oil (sometimes referred to as Palm Christi oil) rendered from the first cold-pressing of the beans is used medicinally. Further pressing yields the grade best suited for soapmaking.

Castor oil's high percentage of *ricinoleic acid,* which gives the oil its high viscosity, sets it apart from all of the other vegetable oils. When calculating the amount of sodium hydroxide required to saponify castor oil, consider the oil's unique makeup. Though it would appear to require less sodium hydroxide, it sometimes requires more, due to its high ricinoleic acid content.

**Use in Soapmaking:**  Like olive oil and jojoba oil, castor oil acts as a humectant by attracting and retaining moisture to the skin. This moisturizing quality makes castor oil well suited for shampoo bars and skin-care products. Castor oil alone is rarely used to make soap because, without other oils, it produces a transparent, soft soap. In combination with other vegetable oils, however, it makes a wonderfully emollient, hard bar of soap.

### COCOA BUTTER

**Nature/Benefits:**  One sniff of a good-quality cocoa butter lets you know that it is obtained from the very same bean as chocolate and cocoa. The butter is pressed from cocoa beans as a by-product of the making of chocolate. Though some people are allergic to cocoa butter, those who

**CAUTION**

Though I like the smell of refined castor oil, it has a stronger odor than other vegetable oils. When it comes time to scent a batch of soap containing a high percentage of castor oil, know that the castor oil will overpower your essential oils. The final bars will not necessarily smell of castor oil, but they will carry a diluted, altered form of your chosen scent. You can protect against this problem by simply keeping the amount of castor oil in your formula in balance. Also, raw castor oil has a protein which is a poison. Be sure to buy detoxified castor oil.

aren't benefit from its moisturizing qualities. It is not easily absorbed by the skin, and it is a very hard, saturated fat, so use it along with more easily absorbed unsaturated oils such as olive, jojoba, castor, or avocado. Cocoa butter lays down a protective layer that holds moisture to the skin, making it a good skin softener. The purest cocoa butter has a strong chocolate scent (though over time, the scent nearly disappears), so I scent a cocoa butter soap with complementary essential oils, such as Peru balsam or vanilla. Deodorized cocoa butter is also available.

**Use in Soapmaking:** A soap made with too high a percentage of cocoa butter will be hard and prone to cracking. Limit cocoa butter to around 15 percent of your total fats and oils. Use it to counterbalance the stickiness of certain fats such as shea butter and lanolin. The cocoa butter formula for White Chocolate Mousse (see page 31) is one of my favorites.

### COCONUT OIL

**Nature/Benefits:** Coconut oil is a gift. It has changed soapmaking more dramatically than any other vegetable oil, and its discovery has led to higher grade soaps. Even companies manufacturing tallow soaps use about 20 percent coconut oil for its lathering and moisturizing properties. Natural soap manufacturers usually combine it with olive, palm, soy, or castor oils for an all-vegetable soap. I cannot say enough about this oil. It offers all soapmaking blends the missing link. Without its wonderful lathering quality, any formula is lacking.

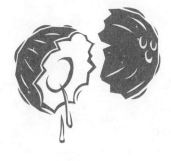

**Types:** Today's soapmaker can purchase coconut oil in a few different phases, each phase with a slightly different melting point: 76°F (24°C), 92°F (33°C), 101°F (38°C), and 110°F (43°C), all available in pails, cubes, or drums. The 76°F (24°C) oil begins to solidify somewhere between 72°F (22°C) and 78°F (26°C); the others solidify around their respective temperatures. The coconut oil found at supermarkets is normally the 76°F (24°C) coconut oil. Soapmakers usually have a preference for a particular phase oil based on their particular methods and formulas.

**Use in Soapmaking:** Coconut oil is obtained from *copra,* which is dried coconut meat. More than any other fat or oil, it is an anomaly. A percentage of coconut oil in cosmetics is moisturizing. Too much of it can be drying. Its saturated nature resists rancidity and makes a very hard soap, yet its low molecular weight allows for high solubility and a quick, fluffy lather, even in cold seawater.

### COTTONSEED OIL

**Nature/Benefits:** Cottonseed oil is a by-product of the cotton industry, obtained by steaming the hulled cottonseeds. Though not as costly as some of the more obscure oils, cottonseed oil normally is too expensive for soapmakers to use in quantity.

**Use in Soapmaking:** Cottonseed oil can be compared to peanut oil with respect to the soap it produces. It is unsaturated, and, though a little slow to saponify with the cold-process, it does offer a quick, abundant, and lasting lather. Cottonseed oil also has emollient qualities, but it is more vulnerable to rancidity than some of the other fats and oils. This is due to a fairly high free fatty acid content, a factor that varies according to the weather endured by the cotton plant after ripening to maturity. Plants exposed to excess rain and humidity render an oil high in free fatty acids and more vulnerable to spoilage. This potential problem can be corrected by reducing the amount of cottonseed oil in your formula.

### EVENING PRIMROSE, BORAGE, AND ROSA MOSQUETA ROSEHIP SEED OILS

**Nature/Benefits:** Evening primrose oil, derived from evening primrose flowers, contains a high content of linoleic acid and, more importantly, gamma-linolenic acid. The small, oval fruit inside the rose bud is called the rose hip, and the oil from one particular species, the Rosa Mosqueta rose, yields an oil rich in essential fatty acids — called Rosa Mosqueta rosehip seed oil. Borage oil, the essential oil derived from the leaves of the borage plant, has even higher percentages of gamma-linolenic acid. The human body does not produce those essential fatty acids (also known as vitamin F), so we must be sure to include those nutrients in our diets and skin-care products.

Essential fatty acids are unique because they offer the skin and the entire body a wide range of benefits. Evening primrose, borage, and Rosa Mosqueta rosehip seed oils are easily absorbed by the skin, encouraging the transport of these essential fatty acids.

### CAUTION

One of my personal concerns with respect to cottonseed oil is today's free use of pesticides by the farming industry. Organic farmers are out there, but very few are growing organic cotton. Most of the cotton grown is sprayed with highly toxic synthetic chemicals, and I have concerns about using its by-products in food and cosmetics.

Essential fatty acids inhibit bacterial growth and encourage the production of antibodies, enabling our systems to defend against infection and inflammation. They also combine with protein and cholesterol to build membranes which link cells to one another. Water loss, resulting in eczema, hair loss, and dry skin, is thought to be related in part to low levels of essential fatty acids. Vegetable oils with high percentages of essential fatty acids ease inflammation and itching, moisturize the skin and scalp, and treat scaly skin and dandruff. These three oils are best suited to dry skin and shouldn't be used by people with oily complexions.

**Use in Soapmaking:** A little goes a long way, though, so each of these oils can be added as superfatting nutrients (1⅔ tablespoons per 5 pounds of soap) just before adding the essential oils.

### HAZELNUT OIL

**Nature/Benefits:** Hazelnut oil is relatively new as a soapmaking oil. It can be derived from many species of the hazelnut tree and is a wonderful moisturizer in creams, lip balms, and soap, since it is absorbed easily by the skin. This oil is unusual in that only two fatty acids account for 90 percent of its fatty-acid content, and both of these are unsaturated. With nearly 80 percent oleic acid and 10 percent linoleic acid, hazelnut oil is one of the most highly unsaturated vegetable oils.

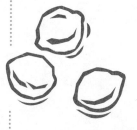

**Use in Soapmaking:** Be sure to include more saturated fats and oils in any soap formula that contains hazelnut oil, for more normal tracing times. With only 7 percent saturated fatty acids, hazelnut oil is in no hurry to saponify.

### HEMP SEED OIL

**Nature/Benefits:** Hemp seed oil is derived from the seed of the plant *Cannabis sativa,* best known as the marijuana plant, and least known for its many productive uses. The hemp plant was banned in the United States in 1937, though it is still legally grown commercially in Europe, Russia, India, and China. Because of hemp's commercial and environmental potential as an economical source of paper, fabric, and fuel, Canada has approved experimental hemp fields — the first since hemp prohibition.

Some activists believe that hemp was banned because it was threatening the potential of the wood industry and the synthetic fiber industry. They claim that those corporations with a stake in the demise of the hemp industry engaged in a smear campaign against hemp. "Hempsters" are those people in the movement who work to educate the public in an effort to bring the hemp plant and its many uses to this country.

Politics aside, hemp appears to offer remarkable benefits. One acre of hemp can yield four times more paper than one acre of trees, for use in newspaper, cardboard, toilet paper, canvas, tampons, stationery and envelopes, and computers. Hemp fiber is much stronger than cotton and produces quality clothing; unlike cotton, it does not demand warm climates with much rainfall. Hemp can grow to 10–20 feet (3–6 m) in height within four months on farmland, at which time it is ready to be harvested, whereas trees require much more land and twenty to fifty years to reach harvest maturity. Cotton growers use pesticides liberally, but hemp has few insect and weed problems, requiring less chemical intervention. Hemp generates more biomass than any of the plants grown here in the United States, and can be converted into a clean, renewable source of energy.

**Types/Availability:** Hemp seed oil can be used as either a primary or a secondary soapmaking oil, though its cost is discouraging. Supply and demand dictate pricing and availability. Since hemp cannot legally be grown in the United States, the supply of its oil is low, and the price high. This price will remain high until either hemp's local growth is legalized or its broad utility is so well understood that more importers choose to carry it.

In the interest of strictly controlling marijuana production in the United States, importing viable seed is illegal. Only sterilized hemp seed that cannot germinate can be purchased by oil manufacturers in this country. It is not clear whether the high temperature of the sterilization process affects the integrity of the essential fatty acid content in hemp seed oil, because the industry is only a few years old and data is not yet available. Some testing suggests that because the seeds are not exposed to heat for extended periods of time, their essential fatty acids are not destroyed. By cold-pressing the sterilized seed using a nitrogen press in an oxygen-free environment, and by keeping the resulting oil in a dark, cool environment away from air, the oil's integrity seems to be maintained.

Some people wonder whether hemp seed oil has any of the intoxicating properties of the leaves. It does not. These properties are derived from a compound called tetrahydrocannabinol (THC), found in the resin in the flowering part of the hemp plant before the seeds are mature enough to be harvested. By the time the seeds are ripe, resin production is low. It is thought that by the time the seeds are cleaned and washed for pressing, they contain no signs of THC.

Some companies purchase the oil from other countries instead of expressing their own from sterilized seed. The owners of Living Seed Products have their hemp grown in Chile, where the viable seeds are cold-pressed using a nitrogen press. They add pure essential rosemary oil in place of any synthetic preservatives, and sell perhaps one of the freshest oils available in the United States, with unaffected essential fatty acids, enzymes, and vitamins E and A. Without empirical data, we must rely upon those in the field using hemp seed on a daily basis. Some of these people feel that the oil expressed from viable seed has a longer shelf life than the oil expressed from sterilized seed. However, local companies that import their hemp seed oil must be conscientious about hands-on management. Foreign hemp seed oil may be better for soap, but since its production takes place out of sight, there is concern about the humanity of foreign labor practices. The folks at Living Seed Products hope to one day be in a position to grow their hemp locally and express their own oil from viable seed; for now, they take pride in closely monitoring the work being done for them out of this country.

**Use in Soapmaking:** Hemp seeds produce a vegetable oil that is high in protein and can be used within a variety of foods and cosmetics. Food-grade, cosmetic-grade, and industrial-grade oils are available. The food-grade oil is the only hemp seed oil pressed in an oxygen-free environment, and therefore better resists oxidation. But because of their high linoleic and linolenic fatty-acid contents, all grades of hemp seed oil are vulnerable to spoilage. Both the food-grade and the cosmetic-grade oils are expensive, but the cosmetic-grade is less costly and fine for soapmaking. Both are cold-pressed without the use of solvents. Avoid bleached hemp seed oil; some bleaching is done to hide rancidity.

The purest hemp seed oil is cold-pressed from viable seed, exposed to minimal heat, light, and oxygen, grown without pesticides and herbicides, and stored at 40–45°F (4.4–7.2°C) temperatures in opaque containers. An oil obtained under these conditions contains essential fatty acids, vitamins, and enzymes that are easily absorbed by the skin and contribute moisturizing qualities to cosmetics and soap. Hemp seed oil is thought to soothe and heal dry skin and minor burns.

Physically, hemp seed oil resembles linseed oil, and its high linoleic and linolenic acid contents make it vulnerable to spoilage. Alpha linolenic, linoleic, and oleic acids — the essential fatty acids known as the omegas — make up 88 percent of the total fatty-acid content. It is the most unstable oil I have ever worked with and yet I consider hemp seed oil worth the fuss. Its instability is a blessing as well as a scourge; it is reactive and more vulnerable to rancidity because it contains the most fragile and the most beneficial fatty acids — the essential fatty acids.

Hemp seed oil requires cool, dark, oxygen-free storage conditions. An unopened container can be stored in the deep freezer indefinitely, and in the refrigerator for a year; an opened container will last for ten to twelve weeks in the refrigerator; and at room temperature, an unopened container can last four to six weeks. An opened container should be used within one to two weeks.

Because of its highly unsaturated nature, I take no more than a 10 percent sodium hydroxide discount when I use hemp seed oil, as 20 to 30 percent of my total soapmaking oils; too much of this free oil in a bar of soap would spoil the bar in a hurry. Though hemp seed oil can be a little stubborn about saponifying, it does just fine in almost any formula. To ensure a hard bar, and to delay rancidity, incorporate saturated fats and oils into a hemp seed oil formula. This is my favorite of all of the soapmaking oils that have come my way in the last couple of years.

### KUKUI NUT OIL

**Nature/Benefits:** The kukui nut tree is the official state tree of Hawaii. Within its fruit are the nuts and kernels from which kukui nut oil is expressed. For hundreds of years, Hawaiians have used this nongreasy oil to treat sunburns and chapped skin. Kukui nut oil is high in linoleic and linolenic acids — essential fatty acids which are critical for healthy skin — and is easily absorbed by the skin. Research has shown kukui nut oil to benefit acne, eczema, psoriasis, sunburn, and chapped skin.

**Use in Soapmaking:** Kukui nut oil is expensive, but a little goes a long way. Even 1⅔ tablespoons added to 5 pounds of soap just before incorporating the essential oils adds richness to your soaps. A higher percentage of kukui nut oil — 10 to 20 percent of the total fats and oils — makes an outstanding soap.

### LANOLIN

**Nature/Benefits:** Lanolin is a fatlike substance (though chemically a wax) produced by the oil glands in sheep and obtained from the sheep's wool. It is used as an emulsifier and an emollient in creams and lotions. It can also be used as an effective emollient in soapmaking formulas. Lanolin is known to effectively soften dry, chapped, cracked skin, as its thick, sticky consistency allows it to remain on the skin longer than many other emollients and therefore hold moisture to the skin for longer periods of time. It is easily absorbed by the skin, adding to its effectiveness. I find lanolin too thick for most applications, however, and I limit its percentage within a soap formula to 2 to 4 percent of my total fats and oils.

Note that lanolin becomes rancid more quickly than other waxes, such as jojoba wax, which never seems to experience rancidity. I refrigerate lanolin for a longer shelf life. Shea butter and lanolin can add stickiness to creams and soaps if you use too high a percentage. Be sure to include saturated fats such as cocoa butter or hydrogenated coconut oil for a smooth finish. Also, consider that lanolin is a common skin sensitizer for some people, sometimes causing allergic reactions. From the time I was little, I detested those beautiful woolen skirts and suits that my mom loved so and urged me to wear. Even a silk slip couldn't distract me from the scratchy, rough feel of the wool. Yet I have no allergy to lanolin. Just be aware that approximately .01 percent of the U.S. population is thought to have allergic reactions to lanolin.

**Use in Soapmaking:** One tablespoon (15 ml) of lanolin per 1 pound (453.6 g) of soap can be added to the melting fats before you add the lye.

### LARD

**Nature/Benefits:** Lard is obtained by rendering and refining the fat of hogs. Most of us don't understand clearly the distinction between the grades of lard, though the characteristics of the soaps each produces differ enough to make it worth our attention. It's more difficult to place orders for fats and oils if we don't really understand how each one works in our soap formulas.

**Types:** Higher grades of lard are edible; lesser grades are inedible. Both are used in soapmaking, though the inedible lard is used more often. The finest lard comes from the fat around the kidneys and has a mild odor. The grades of both edible and inedible lards are no longer clearly defined, and classifications vary from company to company. What once were referred to as choice lard, prime steam lard, and leaf lard, are now known by a variety of names.

Inedible lard is often termed *Choice White Grease,* and, though many soapmakers use it, this grease is associated more with lower grades of soap than the higher grade skin-care soaps. They are made from the less desirable packing house products, and may contain either inedible lard or inedible tallow. They are much higher in free fatty acids than edible lard, so chemical preservatives are often added to delay rancidity.

Most of the fat and oil distributors that carry tallow also carry lard. Some meat processing companies sell lard as a by-product of the manufacturing process.

**Use in Soapmaking:** Whichever lard you choose to use, be sure to use it only in combination with some beneficial vegetable oils. Lard will produce a lasting lather, and it does add conditioning and good cleansing qualities, but lard soaps are soft and not easily soluble in cold water. Its skin-care benefits are negligible, and the lower grades produce soaps which, over time, develop a lard odor. Do add coconut oil, palm oil, and olive oil to the formula. Better yet, consider the animal rights concern, and stick with the multitude of vegetable oils available.

### MACADAMIA NUT OIL

**Nature/Benefits:** Like kukui nut oil, macadamia nut oil is a luxury oil for the soapmaker. Both oils are cold-pressed, highly unsaturated vegetable oils that are easily absorbed into the skin. Macadamia nut oil, also known as Queensland nut oil, comes from the nut of the macadamia tree, a small evergreen tree discovered and named in Australia and planted for industrial use in Hawaii. Macadamia nut oil contains about 80 percent monounsaturated fatty acids and a higher percentage of palmitoleic acid than other vegetable oils. Some studies suggest that palmitoleic acid may act as an antioxidant, protecting cell membranes from deterioration.

Macadamia nut oil is used in gourmet cooking and also makes an emollient soap. Just as most of us limit purchase of the nuts to special occasions, the oil may be too costly to use regularly. Fortunately, this is a stable oil with a longer shelf life than many other vegetable oils.

## NEEM OIL

**Nature/Benefits:** The leaves and the bark of the neem tree are used to treat a variety of skin disorders. The oil has antiseptic properties and is used to treat dandruff, oily skin, and skin diseases such as scabies; it is also an ingredient in mosquito repellents.

**Use in Soapmaking:** Neem oil can be used as a majority soapmaking oil because it is easy to saponify (with its balanced blend of saturated and unsaturated fatty acids), and because it contributes hardness and conditioning properties to its soaps. Neem oil can account for anywhere between 10 and 40 percent of total fats and oils.

## OLIVE OIL

**Nature/Benefits:** The first cold pressing of the olive yields the highest grade extra virgin and virgin olive oils. These oils are released from the first gentle pressing of the olive fruit, without heat or refinement. Refined grade A olive oil is obtained by exerting more pressure on the fruit that has already been squeezed lightly to produce an extra-virgin grade. Extra-virgin olive oil does not require refinement, but the subsequent pressing for virgin olive oil, though cold pressed, contains a higher percentage of free fatty acids and requires some refining. The final pressings of the olives yield what are called grade B refined olive oil and refined pomace olive oil. Grade B refined olive oil is obtained by solvent (usually hexane) extraction using the fruit residue from earlier pressings. Pomace oil is made using the same olive fruit residue used for grade B oil, but it also makes use of the pits (or pomace) of the olives. Each successive pressing is an inferior food grade to the preceding one, but the final pressings are actually best suited for soapmaking.

In soapmaking, olive oil often has the reputation of being one of the more difficult oils to saponify, but, with some basic understanding of the different grades of olive oil (see below), it is as workable as the other fats and oils. It is one of the vegetable oils I consider indispensable and worth the research.

**Types:** For years I've been told that, with respect to soapmaking, one variety of olive oil is no different from another: their fatty acid structures, their SAP values, their free fatty acid contents, and their iodine values are basically the same. I was told to expect a grade A olive oil, a pomace olive oil, and an extra virgin olive oil to experience the same sort of reaction in the soap pan.

This is just not the case. Within each oil is an unsaponifiable portion. These are the components that don't react with the alkali to form soap. They are thought of as impurities, many of which are removed during the refining process. These unsaponifiables are often overlooked because they're a relatively small percentage of the whole, yet I regard them as a rich source of information about a particular oil, especially each grade of olive oil, because the percentages of unsaponifiables vary greatly from one grade to the next. These unsaponifiables can make one grade of olive oil react very differently from another in the soap pan.

The percentage of unsaponifiables is very high in pomace olive oil, and dramatically lower in a grade A olive oil or an extra virgin olive oil. The unsaponifiables in a pomace olive oil create a thick, waxy, synergistic soup, making the oil more viscous, quick to react, and fast to pull the neutral fats into the soapmaking reaction. They act as a catalyst, getting the reaction going and building up some momentum.

Extra-virgin olive oil is the most desirable grade for the gourmet chef, but grades A and B are best suited to the soapmaker, who uses a high proportion of olive oil (nearly half of the total oils) in a vegetable-based soap. Pomace oil, with the highest percentage of unsaponifiables, pulls the other vegetable oils into the quickest saponification, but often the

**CAUTION**

Watch for adulterated olive oils, where the manufacturer or a distributor has incorporated some cheaper oils to increase profits. An adulterated, name brand olive oil caused me a year of processing problems.

pomace oil produces a darker soap, and sometimes overreacts to other soapmaking ingredients, particularly fragrance oils, and even some pure essential oils. Fragrance oils, which often contain *dipropylene glycol,* or even certain pure essential oils like cassia and clove, can cause any soap formula to begin setting up too quickly in the pan, but the reaction seems exaggerated in formulas using a pomace olive oil.

For a vegetable soap formula incorporating a high percentage of olive oil, my preference is a grade A or a grade B refined olive oil. If you only have easy access to the higher grades, expect a longer saponification time, or, with a pomace olive oil, be prepared to act quickly once the fragrance is added.

**Use in Soapmaking:** Olive oil is a very good moisturizer, not because it has its own healing properties, but because it attracts external moisture, holds the moisture close to the skin, and forms a breathable film to prevent loss of internal moisture. Unlike so many other substances used for this purpose, olive oil does not block the natural functions of the skin while performing its own. The skin is able to continue sweating, releasing sebum, and shedding dead skin. Olive oil, jojoba oil, shea butter, kukui nut oil, and some other natural materials do not inhibit these necessary functions.

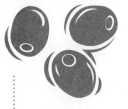

I don't choose my soap's ingredients only for the physical properties they lend to the soap. I want each oil to function also as a skin-care product. For this reason, I use a higher proportion of olive oil and accept its more temperamental nature.

Within the industrial setting, where soaps are often milled, olive oil soaps tend to be very hard. Synthetic additives often contribute to this consistency. For the cold-process soapmaker, olive oil (without synthetic additives) does not make a rock hard soap. You must add coconut and palm oils to ensure a hard bar. The color of the final soap varies with the grade and color of the olive oil used, from white to yellow, from light green to dark green. To make a pure white soap, use a grade A or B refined olive oil that looks bright yellow or gold in the bottle.

Though olive oil soaps produce a slow and stingy lather, they are mild and clean well. Pure olive oil soaps, and those made with a high percentage of olive oil and no harsh additives, are generally safe enough for

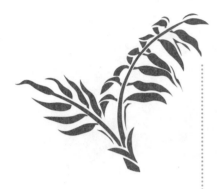

sensitive skin and babies. Castile soap was produced for centuries as 100 percent olive oil soap, though now many companies produce castile bars with part olive oil, part tallow.

### PALM KERNEL OIL AND AMERICAN PALM KERNEL OILS

**Nature/Benefits:** There are many palm kernel oils. The oil obtained from the kernels of the African or oil palm tree is the most familiar; this tree bears the fruit used to make palm oil. The oils obtained from the kernels of Central and South American palm trees yield the American palm kernel oils, including babassu oil.

Palm kernel oil and American palm kernel oils contain large proportions of *lauric acid.* This fatty acid is unusual because it combines two mismatched characteristics: saturation and low molecular weight. These traits enable palm kernel oil, babassu oil, and coconut oil to produce hard soaps that also lather well in all kinds of water. Normally, a saturated fat produces a hard soap with weak lathering ability, but these oils also have low molecular weights, which produce soluble soaps with easy, quick lather. Thus, oils with a high percentage of lauric acid link together the very best of soapmaking characteristics.

**Use in Soapmaking:** Soaps made from either group of palm kernel oils are white, very hard, and lather beautifully. Though some varieties differ with respect to their melting points, this factor is not important to the soapmaker, who only uses a minority percentage of the oil: 10 to 30 percent is plenty when combined with other vegetable oils. This small percentage also keeps the final bars from developing an odor characteristic of the palm kernel oil. Palm kernel oil, like coconut oil, can have a drying effect when used in excess yet is moisturizing when used in moderation.

### PALM OIL

**Nature/Benefits:** Palm oil and palm kernel oil come from one variety of palm tree (the oil palm), while coconut oil comes from another variety (the coconut palm). Palm oil is made from the pulp of the fruit.

**Use in Soapmaking:** A soap made exclusively with palm oil will be brittle and crumble, and, because of its high percentage of free fatty acids, the glycerin yield is low. In many respects, palm oil contributes many of the same qualities as tallow. They both produce a small and slow lather, and their skin-care contribution is negligible.

Palm oil is wonderful, however, within a mixture of other oils. When it is used in combination with olive and coconut oils, it produces a very nice soap. Though coconut oil produces a fluffy, quick lather and makes a hard bar of soap, we must limit its percentage within a formula to avoid a drying effect on skin. This is where palm oil is useful. It, too, makes a hard bar of soap, and, since it is less soluble in water, its firmness holds up throughout use. It also cleans well, saponifies easily, and is mild. Palm oil is the animal rights advocates' substitute for tallow.

My favorite soaps all include some significant portion of palm oil, because it produces hard bars and speeds up the soapmaking process. Palm oil pulls the other soapmaking oils into a quicker saponification. Because the palm oil mixture is more reactive, you must add the essential oils and the nutrients swiftly or the soap will begin to set prematurely.

### PEANUT OIL

**Nature/Benefits:** Peanut oil is made by pressing shelled peanuts. Though considered one of the most important oils in the world, its use in soap should be limited to only a minority percentage of the total oils.

Peanut oil is regarded as a non-drying, conditioning oil, offering the softening qualities of olive and castor oils. It is rich in vitamin E and is absorbed well by the skin. Some soapmakers are experimenting with using it in larger quantities, because it is less expensive in bulk than olive oil, but, for all of its benefits as a straight oil, peanut oil makes soaps that are less than remarkable.

**Use in Soapmaking:** Cold-process soaps made from peanut oil are too soft and produce a stable, but weak and slimy lather. However, the incorporation of palm and coconut oils compensates for its shortcomings. Coconut oil's fluffy, shorter-lived lather, in combination with peanut oil's longer-lasting, fluffless lather, creates a balance. Both coconut and palm ensure harder soaps. Also, like olive oil, peanut oil is highly unsaturated. Soaps containing large proportions of unsaturated oils are more vulnerable to rancidity. Limit the amount of peanut oil to 10 to 20 percent of your total fats and oils.

Once again, maintaining a balance can correct the potential pitfalls of this oil. By all means, experiment with it.

### SAFFLOWER OIL

**Nature/Benefits:** Safflower oil, derived from the seeds of the plant *Carthamus tinctorius,* is used in cosmetics for its moisturizing qualities.

**Use in Soapmaking:** With a higher linoleic-acid content than other oils, safflower oil's shelf life is limited; like hemp seed oil and sunflower oil, it should be used in a soapmaking formula along with saturated fats and oils for harder soap. When you use safflower oil as a majority soapmaking oil, expect slightly longer trace times and a longer cure time to harden the soap. If you have easy, economical access to safflower oil, by all means use it, but expect to accommodate its temperamental nature. It can more easily be used as a minority oil, replacing 10 to 15 percent of another, more costly unsaturated oil.

### SESAME OIL

**Nature/Benefits:** Though new to me as a soapmaking oil, there is nothing new about sesame oil, which has been used for thousands of years. I have always used sesame oil in wok cooking, but only recently have I made soap with it. Sesame oil, like avocado oil and shea butter, contains a high percentage of unsaponifiables (those parts of fats and oils that do not react with sodium hydroxide to form soap and remain in the final bars as conditioning plant nutrients). Sesame oil is used in creams and soaps for its moisturizing qualities, and though some people find that it is more vulnerable to rancidity than other soapmaking oils, none of mine has ever spoiled. This might support some theories that three of its unsaponifiable substances — sesamoline, sesamine, and sesamol — have antioxidant properties that resist rancidity.

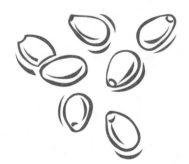

**Use in Soapmaking:** Though I like the strong, nutty smell of sesame oil, many don't. I don't like the smell in soap, however, and it does not take much oil (2 ounces [56.7 g] of sesame oil per 5 pounds [2.3 kg] of soap) to overpower an entire batch. When using a meaningful percentage of the oil in a soapmaking formula, scent the soap with complementary essential oils (see chapter 6). Purchase deodorized sesame oil to avoid the odor completely. With high percentages of oleic and linoleic fatty acids, a sesame oil soap formula should incorporate coconut oil and palm oil for a quicker saponification and a harder bar.

### SHEA BUTTER

**Nature/Benefits:**  Shea butter, also known as African karite butter, is expressed from the pits of the fruit of the African butter tree which grows in Central Africa. This butter has been used for foot and body care. It is remarkably high in unsaponifiables, up to 11 percent, making it a superior superfatting material for soapmaking. Unsaponifiables are those components within the fat or oil which do not decompose and combine with the sodium hydroxide to form soap, thus remaining in their original state within the bars, able to moisturize and nourish the skin.

**Use in Soapmaking:**  Melt the shea butter (2 to 5 percent of your total fats and oils) with the other solid fat. To superfat with shea butter add 1⅔ tablespoons per 5 pounds of soap, melted and cooled to approximately 75°F (24°C) just before adding the scent.

### SOYBEAN OIL (VEGETABLE SHORTENING)

**Nature/Benefits:**  Soybean oil is the primary ingredient in vegetable shortening. It is extracted from the seeds both by pressing and solvent extraction. It contains high percentages of *linoleic* and *oleic acids,* yielding a fairly soft soap, even in the hydrogenated state.

**Use in Soapmaking:**  Though vegetable shortening is often chosen as a nonanimal alternative to tallow or lard, it should be used as a minority oil in combination with oils which offer better skin-care properties. Since it is easy to find and relatively inexpensive, vegetable shortening can be used to contribute bulk, mildness, and a stable lather. Use it in combination with coconut oil for a fluffy lather, and with olive oil for skin conditioning.

### SUNFLOWER OIL

**Nature/Benefits:**  Many soapmakers use sunflower oil as a less expensive alternative to olive oil. It is obtained from the seeds of large sunflowers and known to be a moisturizing vegetable oil. It lays down a

slightly oily protective layer on the skin that holds in moisture. Sunflower oil contains tocopherols (vitamin E) — natural antioxidants that resist rancidity. But with its very high linoleic-acid content, and few saturated fatty acids, sunflower oil should not be stored longer than six months.

**Use in Soapmaking:** Sunflower oil and safflower oil have much in common as soapmaking oils. Soap formulas can include a portion of sunflower oil, though be sure to include other more saturated fats and oils for a quicker saponification and, in the case of superfatted soap, a longer shelf life. I recommend limiting sunflower oil to 10 to 15 percent of your total fats and oils. With higher percentages, consider using an electric mixer for quicker, more reliable tracing, and expect the soaps to take slightly longer to harden.

### TALLOW

**Nature/Benefit:** Tallow has been used in soapmaking more than any other fat or oil. It is extracted by melting the solid, white, flaky fat, or *suet,* surrounding the kidneys and loins of cattle, sheep, and horses. Though soaps have been made for thousands of years from scraps of fat and reused drippings, most of the tallow used in soapmaking today is of a higher grade and lighter color.

**Types:** Only the lighter color grades — which come either from edible tallows or from the higher grades of inedible tallow — are recommended for producing a high-grade soap. These contain fewer *free fatty acids.* Most of the fatty acids found in a fat or an oil are attached to a *glycerol molecule,* forming a *triglyceride.* Those fatty acids not bonded to glycerol, but instead existing independently, are known as free fatty acids. They are less stable than the complete triglyceride, and they contribute to rancidity. The higher grades have a smaller percentage of free fatty acids than the lower grades, offering the soapmaker a more reliable material.

The higher grades also have a cleaner odor, though I detect a "meaty" odor while rendering even the finest grades of tallow. I find that even the final soaps made from home-rendered tallow have a meaty odor, making them somewhat difficult to perfume.

To render your own tallow, you'll need to find a meat-packing plant or a good butcher to package the suet for you. For large quantity soap-making, rendering your own tallow is impractical. It requires heating the solid suet with some water and a little salt, eventually yielding cleaner, purer tallow. The process is time-consuming and messy, leaving you with greasy pans and surfaces, even after washing and scouring. It's a bit like plaster dust — it winds up in spots you could swear you were nowhere near. Ann Bramson's book, *Soap: Making It, Enjoying It,* in which she details the rendering process, is a good resource. Try rendering once, but, for long-term soapmaking with tallow, locate a fat manufacturer or distributor that sells pre-rendered tallow in pails.

**Use in Soapmaking:** Quite a bit of controversy surrounds the use of tallow in soapmaking. It is thought to clog pores, cause blackheads, and increase the incidence of eczema for individuals with sensitive skin. Tallow's high molecular weight and saturated structure make an insoluble bar of soap with a weak and slimy, though longer-lasting, lather. Tallow supporters point to the wonderfully hard bars it produces, and its ability to saponify (harden into soap) quickly. It is also relatively inexpensive and plentiful. Supporters cite the 5,000 years of tallow use as evidence that it's safe.

Those who oppose the use of tallow do not deny its value to past centuries; they just question its continued use in light of today's alternatives. Some animal rights advocates distinguish between need and convenience: pioneers would not have been able to keep disease under control without using animal by-products to make soap. Their herbal alternatives were far less effective. Today, we have a smorgasbord of vegetable oils to replace tallow in soaps. Many people consider it immoral to kill an animal for a bar of soap, when so many vegetable oils make worthy substitutes. Others argue that animals are sacrificed for their meat and not their by-products, which would only go to waste without soapmaking and other by-product industries. However, the profitability of selling by-products theoretically subsidizes the sale of meat, permitting lower meat prices and encouraging greater meat consumption.

## HYBRIDIZED OILS

The food industry and the soapmaking industry share an interest in saturated and unsaturated fats and oils. Soapmakers balance saturated and unsaturated fats and oils for the ideal blend of soap characteristics; the food industry uses both saturated and unsaturated fats and oils, though health concerns have buoyed unsaturated fats to prominence, leaving saturated fats relegated to frying, coating, and icing. Saturated coconut and palm oils produce nice hard soaps with generous lathers, but a diet of coconut oil and palm oil contributes to heart disease. In their food, consumers now prefer oils with high percentages of monounsaturates, those unsaturated fatty acids with one double bond (see chapter 13) that are thought to reduce the LDL cholesterol levels while maintaining the level of HDL cholesterol.

### Hybridization

Today's agricultural technology has produced some interesting hybrid seed in an attempt to breed plants and oils that compare favorably to the originals. The food industry has developed high–oleic acid canola and sunflower hybrids to replace the more saturated oils, and a high–lauric acid canola oil to reduce dependence upon imported tropical oils such as coconut and palm kernel. The high–oleic acid oils were created through a series of plant crossings; the laurate canola oil was genetically engineered.

Using selective breeding, two different companies have designed a high–oleic acid sunflower oil and a high–oleic acid canola oil. Plants with varying fatty acid compositions are "mated" to produce new plants (and, ultimately, oils) that have the more desirable fatty-acid composition. Over time, a plant that produces an oil with a meaningful percentage of saturated fatty acids can be developed into a plant whose oil is highly unsaturated.

The technology is fascinating. The same species of plant grown in two different climates may produce oils with slightly different fatty-acid compositions. One may be slightly higher or lower in oleic- and linoleic-acid content. The levels of these two fatty acids are interrelated; often, an increase in one means a decrease in the other. By cross-pollinating plants with sightly different fatty-acid structures in a controlled greenhouse setting, however, hybridized plants with higher monounsaturate levels and lower saturate levels have been created. The vegetable oils produced by these new plants are currently considered healthful alternatives to the more saturated fats and oils of years past.

A different technology, genetic engineering, has developed the hybridized laurate canola oil. A gene from the California bay laurel tree high in lauric acid was inserted into canola seed. The gene, an enzyme, recognizes $C_{12}$ (lauric acid) production and transforms a canola seed without lauric acid into a canola seed with a high lauric-acid content. This genetic manipulation is done in the lab and actually rearranges the DNA of the plant. Scientists literally create a new canola plant whose fatty-acid composition compares favorably with that of coconut oil and palm kernel oil. Though it is too soon to know, preliminary research suggests that laurate canola oil soap may lather better and be more gentle than coconut oil and palm kernel oil soaps. The superior lather may relate to the structured placement of the $C_{12}$ on the triglyceride; the gentleness may be due to the absence of caprilic acid and capric acid — irritating fatty acids found in coconut and palm kernel oils. The development of laurate canola has followed close on the heels of high–oleic acid hybridization, and the new crop is being crushed into oil as I finish this book.

## Hybridized Oils as Soapmaking Oils

Considering the fluctuating costs of olive oil, coconut oil, and palm kernel oil, some soapmakers substitute cheaper oils. The perfect fit is not yet available but, over time, hybridized oils may come closer to our specs.

Laurate canola oil is not yet available, and high–oleic acid oils may be too highly unsaturated to use in high percentages in superfatted formulas. The problem is that high–oleic acid soaps do not saponify as quickly and the final bars take longer to harden. Ridden of saturated fatty acids, these polyunsaturated oils instead contain fatty acids with more than one double bond; these double bonds bend the fatty-acid chains, making it more difficult for lye to reach the bonds and react to form soap. The polyunsaturated oils include safflower, soybean, canola, and sunflower. (Though castor oil is highly unsaturated, it saponifies readily due to its ricinoleic-acid content.) Even olive oil, which can be temperamental because of its unsaturated nature, contains saturated fatty acids and therefore saponifies without difficulty. To avoid long tracing times and longer curing times, keep your percentage of high–oleic acid hybrid oils to 10 to 20 percent of the total fats and oils you use in a formula.

## Innovators

SVO Specialty Products, Inc., in Ohio has produced a line of hybridized, high–oleic acid sunflower oils under the brand name Trisun. They are preserved with natural tocopherols, with neutral flavor and odor. AC Humco recently purchased SVO and now markets this oil. Another company, Cargill Foods, developed its Clear Valley high–oleic acid canola oil from hybridized canola seeds grown in the Pacific Northwest — eastern Washington, Idaho, and Montana. This oil grew out of a project conceived of over a decade ago by E. I. Dupont to study DNA plant technology. Calgene Chemical, Inc., recently harvested the first genetically engineered canola oil in Georgia. Canola oil does not contain laurate triglycerides, but Calgene's creation, laurate canola, contains around 40 percent lauric acid.

The good news is that science continues to create useful materials. The progress seems miraculous and speedy to me, and I suspect that it will not be too long before small soapmakers can purchase these oils in pails. Since hybridized oils are so new to the market, my hunch is that these companies will sell only in drum quantities until they see profit potential in selling the smaller quantities.

**Tocopherols**

A classification in the vitamin E group, tocopherols are fat-soluble antioxidant compounds of vitamin E that are used to preserve soap. Look for the natural tocopherols made from vegetable sources and avoid the synthetic imitations. Note that tocopherols protect tallow and lard soaps better than they protect all-vegetable soaps.

# CHAPTER 5
## Using Natural Colorants

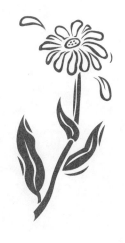

$O$nce you have perfected basic soapmaking formulas, it's fun to experiment with color. Though this step is simple, I encourage beginners to wait until they understand the basics before adding colorants. Beginners improve their skills and come into their own as soapmakers one batch at a time. Because soapmaking involves a chemical reaction, it is — like any other scientific process — most effectively studied in a controlled way. Introducing one or two new ingredients to the equation at a time helps you keep better track of exactly what contributes to varying results. After you understand the basics — temperature, stirring, and the correct balance of raw materials — then the time has come to play with signature bars. Color is a fun toy, but it should come last.

I urge you to resist the temptation to color soaps with RIT dye, food coloring, tempera paints, candle dye, or the minerals that potters use to create ceramic glazes. Fabric dye can be chemically active and is generally considered toxic. Many artists' pigments that are thought to be inert minerals can contain impurities and are sometimes toxic in powdered form. A soap that has been carefully crafted with fine, pure ingredients will be contaminated by this one final splash of color. But a bright yellow that comes from annatto seed, or a seafoam green from spirulina, contributes color while preserving the integrity of the soap.

Whenever I'm tempted to make a dark red, a burgundy, or a black soap from the various iron oxides, I remind myself of my original goal: to control what goes into my soap. Common sense guides us fairly well. If we have a hunch that RIT dye doesn't belong in soap, then it probably doesn't. If innocuous plant seeds, roots, or leaves contribute color, and this offering seems a healthful, stable alternative, then it probably is. Resist the temptation to over-orchestrate color using any and all possibilities.

# AN OVERVIEW OF COLORANTS

Colorants are the substances included in a soap formula to produce color in the final bars. It is worthwhile to distinguish between a dye and a pigment, both of which are colorants.

Dyes are water-soluble substances that lend color to a material by combining molecularly with it. In a part-chemical, part-physical union, the colored dye enters the fibers and fixes to them. If a dye is resistant to light and does not bleed into the soap lather, it is considered colorfast.

Pigments are usually colored or white compounds that are soluble neither in the material to which they lend color nor in water. Pigments do not react chemically — their physical compositions do not change within the material they dye, in this case soap. Instead they scatter throughout the soap and absorb and reflect light. Pigments can be inorganic or organic, natural or synthetic, and they are fairly stable once dispersed and immobilized in the soap. Inorganic pigments include ultramarines, iron oxides, bronze powder, chromium oxide greens and white, titanium dioxide, barium sulfate, zinc oxide, sienna, and ochers.

## Natural versus Synthetic Colorants

Many people experience mild to severe reactions to synthetic colorants such as coal-tar dyes and various pigments. Even small amounts of these allergens will cause itching, rashes, and inflammation. But natural colorants are not all perfect angels.

Minerals and clays mined from the earth are often filled with impurities. The FDA disallows the use of natural iron oxide in cosmetics because of the high level of heavy metals (mercury, lead, and arsenic) discovered in nearly all samples tested by x-ray scanning. The soapmaker is often exempt from these rules, since some soap is not subject to federal regulation (see chapter 17, page 270). Still, if the FDA disallows certain colorants in cosmetics, shouldn't the soapmaker wonder why?

Natural is not always better. There are many natural colorants that are either mildly irritating, questionable, or absolutely dangerous to use in a skin-care product. Many dye plants contain some sensitizers and toxins, and the factor determining toxicity is often the percentage of colorant used in a formula. A synthetic ultramarine, found in minute amounts in bars of soap, may be safer to use than a natural color from plants such as tansy or logwood. A list of unsafe skin-care colorants — which would include fabric and candle dyes, potters' minerals, and oil paints — would be incomplete without the inclusion of certain plant colorants used in certain quantities.

Unfortunately, these quantities are as yet undetermined. Many of the suspect plants lead double lives. Like many of the pure essential oils, and some of the seemingly harmless foods and drinks that we consume, these plants appear to be nontoxic in small quantities and dangerous in excess. All of the chemists I have spoken to feel that the anthraquinones in madder root that are carcinogenic are most likely harmless in the minute quantities found in final bars of soap. Interestingly, some studies suggest that small doses of anthraquinones prevent certain cancers, while other studies show that larger doses cause cancers. It is not unusual for the chemicals in plants to be both beneficial and lethal, depending upon usage.

Research each potential colorant on a case-by-case basis. Should the synthetic version be questionable, do not fall back on the natural version unless it is considered safe. Should a natural colorant be worrisome, do not settle for an unproven synthetic version. Natural is not always better than synthetic. Sometimes, consider using neither.

And remember that color rarely improves a soap. It is fun and eye-catching, but it seldom creates a better product. Unless you are comfortable with a colorant, avoid it and let the soapmaking ingredients tint the soap naturally.

## Take Nothing for Granted: Experiment!

The chemistry of dye plants, the chemistry of soapmaking, and the chemistry of the dye process must be completely understood for failure-free experimentation. We should all expect to be surprised — and often. Our best discoveries are the result of trial and error. This is how I learned that alkanet root colors a more alkaline solution blue and a slightly less alkaline solution purple; that the addition of alcohol turns a blue solution purple; that the beautiful magenta of beetroot powder turns muddy yellow in the presence of lye; that soapwort produces a gorgeous lime green soap on day one — which fades to drab yellow-brown in time; and that the indigo that dyes fabric lovely shades of blue is insoluble in every phase of the soapmaking process.

I can share everything that my experimentation has taught me, but I have only scratched the surface of the possible combinations of color. There remain many more dye plants and many untried soapmaking formulas yet to be widely recognized as soap colorants. Also, the natural shades of the many fats, oils, nutrients, and essential oils used in soap will blend with plant colorants to produce new colors. Finally, using more than one plant colorant at a time — blending colorants — produces the most interesting results.

Keep in mind that all soap colorants are affected differently by heat, light, acidity, and alkalinity. To the extent that your soapmaking process intrudes upon these factors, your final results will be affected. *Most dye plants color a less alkaline soap a different shade, or even a different color completely, than they color a more alkaline soap. The results and procedures described in this chapter relate to less alkaline soap (using my 10 percent discount), not to fully saponified soap.* Enjoy the offshoots you discover and the knowledge that your soap is uniquely yours.

## PLANT COLORANTS AND THE SOAPMAKING PROCESS

Though many plants contain coloring matter, some release their color more readily than others, and some have more color to release. Some are more affected by the alkalinity of the lye, contributing different colors to more alkaline soap mixtures (or vice versa). Some are soluble in water, others in oil or alcohol.

The list beginning on page 124 includes a variety of colorants that can be used in soapmaking. Those that produce the best color most efficiently are discussed in more detail; those less effective are more generally

## SOAPMAKING NOTE: COLORANTS

Often, a wonderful plant colorant is passed over too quickly after a cursory test reveals it less than satisfactory. Before giving up on a plant, test the parts containing the coloring matter in the lye solution, in the melted fats and oils, and in the final soap mixture at the trace. If you tested alkanet root only in the lye solution, you would consider it a dud. But dissolve it in olive oil and it releases a beautiful shade of scarlet.

Explore all possible phases, though keep in mind that some phases are less reliable bets: Large annatto seeds are not added at the trace, for example, since the solid pieces would remain in the final bars; nor are glassy chunks of cutch added at the trace because the last-minute rush would not allow time for the cutch to fully dissolve, leaving sharp pieces in the soap.

To minimize waste, I test a potential colorant three ways before making a larger batch of soap with it. It is better to use more rather than less plant material when testing a colorant; you can always incorporate less of it in your perfected formula if the test shade is too dark or bleeds, but if you use too little, you are likely to discount the plant's usefulness. My test method is described below. Steps 1 and 2 do not require precise measurements; they are designed to 1. let you know whether or not the plant is soluble in a particular phase, and 2. give you a feel for how readily the plant releases its coloring.

Remember that a tiny amount of soap mixture can take longer to trace than a large batch that retains more heat, so use higher-range soapmaking temperatures and stir as quickly as possible. If you don't mind washing the extra dishes, you can let the soap beat away in a freestanding mixer.

▲▲▲▲▲

### Three Steps to Fully Testing a Colorant

1. First, dissolve about a teaspoon (5 ml) of sodium hydroxide into a couple of tablespoons (about 30 ml) water. Then add the plant material (powdered for best release of color) to the lye solution, stirring to release the pigment. Note the resulting color, and the depth of the shade.

2. Next, blend some of the plant material with a small amount of a fatty oil such as olive oil or vegetable oil (heated slightly for greater solubility). Stir well and note the color and depth of the shade.

3. Finally, make *one* bar of soap (see the recipe for the Experimental Bar on page 24) using the colorant in the phase that proved stronger (lye or oil). You can make a second bar if you want to try adding the powdered, coarsely chopped, or whole plant material at the trace. After using a variety of plant colorants, you should have a feel for how much plant material to experiment with per bar. Keep track of the amount used to color the one bar and multiply by 12 for a 5-pound (2.3-kg) batch of soap.

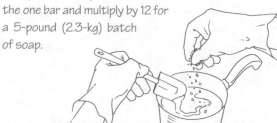

reviewed. For instance, annatto seed produces a richer yellow than nandina berry, goldenrod, or elderberry, and requires far less plant material to achieve the deeper shades, so it is described thoroughly. Still, while you may be tempted to choose the colorant with more bang for the buck, enjoy experimenting with a wide range of nature's offerings. The colorants listed and described without instructions for use are those known to be safe dye plants that I have not yet used myself.

### ALKANET ROOT *(Alkanna tinctoria)*

**Nature:** This biennial or perennial has bright blue flowers and a thick red-maroon taproot that releases a rich, dark red dye in alcohol or oil, and a less intense shade in boiling water. Historically, the root was ground and used as a face rouge. Alkanet root steeped in oil makes an imitation rosewood or mahogany wood stain. Medicinally, alkanet root is used as an astringent, and for its antimicrobial properties.

Alkanet root contains alkannin, a naphthoquinone, which is part of the family of anthraquinones (see "Madder Root"). Many studies suggest that the naphthoquinones in alkanet root contain antimicrobial and wound-healing properties. Like the related anthraquinones, naphthoquinones may be carcinogenic when used in certain concentrations. A lack of data relating to alkanet root and its use as a cosmetic colorant, however, leaves us to piece together the fragmented and sometimes conflicting findings. My hunch is that alkanet and madder root, when used in the small quantities described in this book, probably pose no risk. But I repeat the need to exercise judgment and caution.

**Quantity/Procedure:** Alkanet root is an herbal version of a pH test, somewhat like the litmus plant. It colors an acid vegetable oil with a pH of 6 red, a somewhat alkaline soap mixture with a pH of 8 shades of lavender, and a more alkaline soap mixture with a pH of 10 shades of blue. The concentration of alkanet in the solution affects the depth of the shade. Depending upon the alkalinity of the soap and the concentration of the alkanet root, the lavender colors it produces can vary from gray-lavender to deep lavender to purple, and its blue can range from faded pastel blue to robin's-egg blue to dark blue.

## UNDERSTANDING pH

pH measures the acidity of a substance in solution. A substance dissolved in water that increases the hydrogen ion concentration of the solution is an acid (below 7 on the pH scale). A substance dissolved in water that increases hydroxyl (or the hydroxide) ion (OH⁻) concentration of the solution is a base (above 7 on the pH scale). The higher the pH, the lower the concentration of hydrogen ions, and therefore the less acidic the substance is.

To use alkanet root as a soap colorant, replace a portion of your soap-making oils with an equal portion of colored, strained alkanet oil. To make the alkanet oil for a 5-pound (2.3-kg) batch of soap, add ¾ cup (175 ml) cut and sifted alkanet root to 1 cup (250 ml) olive oil, or whichever unsaturated oil is most predominant in the formula you want to color purple (or blue, if your soap is more alkaline). Stir the mixture to release some of the dark red color into the oil. Let it steep for a period of hours, stirring periodically to release more color. Strain before using.

For shades of darker purple (in less alkaline soap) or blue (in more alkaline soap), replace 1 cup (250 ml) of the unsaturated soapmaking oils with the 1 cup (250 ml) strained alkanet oil *before* you pour the lye into the fats and oils. For lavender or light blue, replace only 4 tablespoons (60 ml) of the soapmaking oils with only 4 tablespoons (60 ml) of alkanet oil.

### ANNATTO SEED (*Bixa orellana*)

**Nature:** This small flowering shrub grows in Central America and has large, pink flowers that look like roses. A red coloring made from the pulp around the seeds of this plant was used by the Mayan civilization as a dye. The seeds and pulp are separated from the remainder of the fruit, and the pulp is crushed in water, strained, and finally pressed into annatto beads. These dried, red beads contain the carotenoid bixin, which, in the presence of a base, turns shades of orange and yellow. This range of color is lent to soap when annatto is used as a colorant.

When the red wax is extracted from the annatto seed using organic solvents, the resulting product is called bixin; when it is extracted using potassium or sodium hydroxide, it is called norbixin. For those who want to avoid steeping annatto seeds in vegetable oil for a colored oil, two forms of concentrated ready-to-use annatto are available: Water-soluble powdered annatto, called norbixin, and oil-soluble bixin extract. I prefer either the oil-soluble annatto seed or the oil-soluble bixin extract to the water-soluble powder.

**Quantity/Procedure:** Though not as colorfast as some dyes, annatto produces gorgeous, rich shades of yellow and orange. Keep the soap away from direct sunlight to prevent fading. To use annatto beads as a

**ADDING COLORANT TO LYE**

Whenever you add plant material to a lye solution, be sure to add it to freshly made, hot lye for the fullest release of color. Steep for at least thirty minutes — preferably for an hour or two.

colorant, prepare an annatto oil (similar to alkanet oil, described on preceding page). To color 15 pounds (6.8 kg) of soap a deep shade of orange- yellow, add 3⅓ tablespoons plus 2 teaspoons (62.5 ml) annatto seed to ¾ cup (175 ml) olive oil (or the liquefied oil of your choice). Heat the oil slightly before leaving it to steep for an hour or so, stirring occasionally to release more color. Strain the annatto oil; then use it to replace an equal portion of your other melted fats and oils.

To produce a butter yellow color, add 1½ tablespoons (22.5 ml) annatto seeds per ½ cup (125 ml) olive or jojoba oil. Heat on high in the microwave for thirty seconds; then let the mixture rest for an hour or so, stirring occasionally to release more color. For a 5-pound (2.3-kg) batch of soap, replace 5 tablespoons plus 2 teaspoons (85 ml) of liquid vegetable oils with this *strained* annatto oil just before adding the lye solution.

Dissolve ¼–½ teaspoon (1–2.5 ml) powdered annatto (per 5 pounds [2.3kg] of soap) into the freshly mixed lye solution for varying shades of orange. *Note:* Too much powder bleeds into the lather.

For yellows and oranges, add anywhere from a few drops to ½ teaspoon (2.5ml) of oil-soluble bixin extract (per 5 pounds [2.3 kg] soap) to the soapmaking oils before adding the lye, or to the soap at trace (less for yellows, more for oranges). I prefer to add the extract at the trace.

### BEETROOT POWDER *(Beta vulgaris)*

**Nature:** Beetroot powder is made by dehydrating mature beets and then processing the roots into a purplish red powder. Beetroot powder contains red and yellow pigments and colors soap an earthy squash yellow — a darker, muddier shade of what turmeric produces in soap.

**Quantity/Procedure:** Note that the smell of beetroot is strong and lasting; you will want to scent your soap sufficiently when using this colorant. For a 5-pound (2.3-kg) batch of soap, whisk 2 tablespoons (30 ml) beetroot powder into the lye solution, strain, and add to the fats and oils; then add 1½ tablespoons (22.5 ml) beetroot powder at the trace (first whisking it into ½ cup [125 ml] of the soap mixture, then adding this colored soap back into the rest of the soap).

## BETA-CAROTENE

**Nature:** Carotenoids are the orange or red coloring compounds found in plants and in some animal tissues. Beta-carotene is one of these provitamin-A constituents found in carrots, butter, and egg yolks, extracted as red crystals or crystalline powder and used by some soap-makers to produce shades of yellow-orange. Beta-carotene is thought to be an antioxidant and to treat acne.

**Quantity/Procedure:** Unrefined palm oil contains beta-carotene and produces yellow to red shades, depending upon the blend of soapmaking fats and oils. Pure beta-carotene can be added to soap (⅛ teaspoon [.6 ml] per 12 pounds [5.4 kg] of soap, dissolved first in a little water) just before you pour it into a mold. Oil-soluble beta-carotene extract is added to the fats and oils, or at the trace. Most of the beta-carotene available today is synthetic, and the naturally derived material is exorbitantly expensive, so I recommend annatto instead as a source for yellow and orange.

## BLACK-EYED SUSAN *(Rudbeckia hirta)*

**Nature:** This easy-to-grow, prolific perennial (sometimes a biennial) blooms for months and produces tough stems and flower heads with yellow petals and brown-black centers. The leaves and stems produce gold-orange tones, and the flower heads produce olive green or brown-ish green tones.

**Quantity/Procedure:** Add ¾ cup (175 ml) finely chopped fresh yellow petals to the lye solution, strain, and add to the fats and oils. The dark orange lye solution will fade to a soft yellow in your final bars.

## BRAZILWOOD *(Caesalpinia vidacea)*

**Nature:** There are nine varieties of the redwood tree that produce the true brazilwood sawdust used as a red dye. The sawdust releases more color than do brazilwood chips.

**Quantity/Procedure:** To color soap an antique pink-mauve shade, powder the sawdust and steep approximately 2 tablespoons (30 ml) of it in the lye solution for every 5 pounds (2.3 kg) of soap. Strain the lye solution before adding it to the fats and oils.

## CALENDULA BLOSSOMS *(Calendula officinalis)*

**Nature:** Calendula was once referred to as pot marigold, though it does not belong to the Tagetes family.

**Quantity/Procedure:** Pale yellow and deep orange calendula blossoms contribute yellow-orange tones to soap, somewhat as safflower does. The blossoms are a little stingy with their color, so I grind them into a powder for more of it, but also add the long fibers for texture and beauty. Add at the trace approximately 2 tablespoons (30 ml) of the powder and 1 tablespoon (15 ml) of the fibers per pound of soap.

## CHLOROPHYLL

**Nature:** Chlorophyll is the bright green pigment found in the chloroplasts of plants. This pigment absorbs light energy, which initiates photosynthesis and converts chlorophyll into sugars. Chlorophyll consists mainly of two esters (see chapter 13, "The Chemistry of Soapmaking"): a blue-black one ($C_{55}H_{72}O_5N_4Mg$), and a dark green one ($C_{55}H_{70}O_6N_4Mg$). Chlorophyll, a microcrystalline wax, is used as a deodorizing agent and a green colorant. It is soluble in fats and alcohol but not in water (only synthetic chlorophyll can be dissolved in water).

Soapmakers can purchase chlorophyll in different forms: liquid (often synthetic), natural powder, and synthetic powder (see "Suppliers" in the appendix).

*Liquid Chlorophyll (part synthetic).* Liquid chlorophyll is often sodium copper chlorophyllin (not natural) mixed with water. When added just before the trace, liquid chlorophyll tints the soap a lovely pale green. Darker greens are tough to achieve at this stage of the soapmaking process because too much liquid will overload the soap and precipitate out of solution. For dark green shades, you can instead replace most to all of the water with liquid chlorophyll, dissolving the sodium hydroxide in the liquid chlorophyll.

*Water-Soluble Powder, Sodium Copper Chlorophyllin (part synthetic).* Sodium copper chlorophyll contains natural chlorophyll, but is produced synthetically. This water-soluble powder is a bright, intense green, and — depending upon how much is used — colors soap light green to a deep, bright forest green. The natural base for this synthetic powder consists of chlorophyll extracted from alfalfa, spinach, and mulberry leaves. The chlorophyll is split by hydrolysis, and part of its ester group is replaced by sodium or potassium. Copper is also added to the group, and the resulting salt is called a chlorophyllin. It is water-soluble. Sodium copper chorophyllin contributes a beautiful shade of green to cold-process soap but unfortunately is vulnerable to spoilage, and not only in the presence of light. My hunch is that the synthetic manipulation of the chlorophyll leaves the resulting arrangement less stable. As the chlorophyll breaks down, the soap begins to brown around the edges and smell rancid.

*Oil-Soluble Powder (natural).* Most natural chlorophyll colorants are extracted from alfalfa or spinach as an oily paste. For deeper greens, around 2 percent of this natural chlorophyll paste (straight chlorophyll) is added to around 1 to 2 percent powdered chlorophyll from spray-dried alfalfa. Though the chlorophyll from plants is oil soluble, when it is complexed in the plant with other water-soluble plant components, the chlorophyll becomes slightly water soluble. But the added 2 percent straight chlorophyll is oil soluble, creating a final natural chlorophyll that is more oil soluble than water soluble, and better incorporated into the soap than into the lye solution.

**Quantity/Procedure:** Liquid chlorophyll is added either at the trace or as a replacement for all or part of the water (4 tablespoons [60 ml] at the trace per 5 pounds [2.3 kg] of soap, or up to the total percentage of the water as a replacement). You will achieve less color if you add it at the trace, because the soap mixture cannot accommodate more than a few extra tablespoons of liquid at this point. If you choose to replace the water, add the sodium hydroxide to the liquid chlorophyll just as you would add it to plain water. You can achieve deeper colors with powdered sodium copper chlorophyllin than you can with liquid, though, so why pay for water? The liquid is less economical, and now that I know that it, too, is synthetic, I find no compelling reason to choose it over the powdered form.

Dark green oil-soluble chlorophyll powder has a heavy, sticky consistency. Around 1½ teaspoons (7 ml) of powder per 5 pounds (2.3 kg) of soap colors the soap a beautiful shade of avocado green. Add the powder

**BE AWARE OF PLANTS' POWERS**

Just because something is natural does not mean that it is always mild. Modern life exposes us to many potentially toxic, natural chemicals — from our air-conditioning and swimming pools to our vegetables, fruits, laxatives, coffee, and tea. It's difficult to find a plant lacking the chemicals that in a given situation, and a given quantity, are toxic to something or someone. Many effective chemicals are both safe and unsafe. For example, the tannic acid found in walnuts, sumac, Saint-John's-wort, cutch, henna, coffee, and tea is used safely as an astringent and to treat burns; in excess, however, it causes irritation and alters pigmentation. Most plants have a dark side when used incorrectly but make meaningful contributions in moderation.

to a cup (250 ml) of saponified soap; then add this mixture back into the rest of the saponified soap. Scent and pour.

Water-soluble chlorophyll powder offers the brightest, clearest shades of green. Very little is required for gorgeous color; just a few grains of the powder turns water bright emerald green. For a bright forest green color, add ¼ teaspoon (1 ml) of the water-soluble powder per 5 pounds (2.3 kg) soap. For a lighter green, add a small pinch (about ½₄ teaspoon [.2 ml]) of the water-soluble powder per 5 pounds (2.3 kg) soap.

### CINNAMON *(Cinnamomum zeylanicum, Cinnamomum cassia)*

**Nature:** This tropical evergreen tree has fragrant, thick bark and leaves, along with oval, bluish fruit. The bark is used medicinally as an antiseptic, astringent, and stimulant.

**Quantity/Procedure:** Ground cinnamon powder contributes warm brown shades and speckles to soap. Too much cinnamon can make the final soap scratchy, but a lighter sprinkling adds a warm, spicy appeal.

### COCHINEAL *(Dactylopius coccus)*

**Nature:** Cochineal is a natural red dye obtained from the dried bodies of a female beetle that feeds on cacti in Mexico and Central America. Seventy thousand dried cochineal beetles are required to produce 1 pound (.45 kg) of dye, and 200,000 pounds (90,720 kg) of beetles can be harvested from one acre of land. They are killed by immersion in scalding water or by drying them in ovens or in the sun. Though once relied upon heavily for crimson shades, cochineal has been replaced as a common red dye by synthetic azo dyes.

**Quantity/Procedure:** If you use cochineal to color soap, you must add it at the trace to achieve magenta tones. Adding it to the lye solution turns the soap a different color completely — a pretty, pale mauve-pink. Some consumers are unfazed to learn that the beautiful magenta color of their skin-care products is a powdered insect; but I think that many people find this option distasteful. Our only gain from it is aesthetic, and we have many other choices, so I cannot find my way to cochineal. Without debating human versus animal versus insect sacrifice, I cannot help but wonder what beautiful shade some part of me might contribute.

### COCOA *(Theobroma cacao)*

**Nature:**  Cocoa, made from the roasted seeds of the cacao plant, is a ground powder with a bitter chocolate scent.

**Quantity/Procedure:**  You can use cocoa as a warm brown colorant, either for solid color or for marbling. Before choosing it over one of the other brown colorants, however, note that some people are allergic to cocoa in food and in skin-care products. Also, too much cocoa leaves a soap with an odd smell that overpowers your chosen scent.

To use cocoa as a colorant, whisk it into a small amount of traced soap, then add this darker soap back into the rest of the mixture. Marbled brown-and-white bars can be made by whisking 2 teaspoons (10 ml) cocoa into 2 cups (500 ml) of lightly traced soap, then marbling the darker soap into the remaining soap in your mold.

### COMFREY ROOT AND LEAF *(Symphytum officinale)*

**Nature:**  The leaves and the root of this herbaceous perennial are used medicinally to heal and soothe. The mucilage and the allantoin in comfrey root are the principal constituents contributing to its use as a demulcent, an astringent, and an expectorant. Comfrey is also thought to regenerate cell growth after injury. Comfrey leaves are used externally to treat swelling, sprains, and bruises.

**Quantity/Procedure:**  The root can be ground and used to color soap a deep sage green (2 tablespoons [30 ml] per 5 pounds [2.3 kg] of soap). My friend Terrianne Taylor suggests soaking dried comfrey leaves before incorporating them in soap, for green specks. (After many weeks, the herbs eventually fade to brown.) Prepare an herbal infusion using dried comfrey and let the mixture sit in the refrigerator for a few days. Just before adding the lye to the fats and oils, strain the herbs from the infusion and squeeze them dry. Wrap the herbs in plastic and set them aside until the trace. Then incorporate them into the soap mixture for green specks in your final bars.

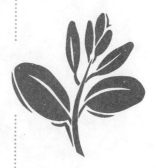

### CUTCH *(Acacia catechu)*

**Nature:**  Cutch, also known as gum arabic, is derived from the dried stem of the mimosa tree. For over 2,000 years, this extract from the wood has been used as a brown dye that is extremely resistant to light. To obtain the extract, the bark is stripped from the cutchwood; then the wood is chopped and simmered in boiling water. The extract that is released during this process is recovered and left to thicken and solidify as it cools.

Cutch is used as a demulcent to soothe irritations, though it causes skin rashes in sensitive individuals. An infusion of catechu is used to stop nosebleeds; the plain powder or an ointment is applied externally to skin eruptions, such as boils and skin ulcers.

**Quantity/Procedure:** You will find cutch in its final form as solid, glassy chunks, brownish black in color. The brittle resin can be broken into small pieces that will better dissolve into the hot lye solution. Mix pieces of cutch with the lye solution just after you add the sodium hydroxide to the water; leave the cutch in the lye (stirring occasionally) until the lye is ready to be poured into the soapmaking oils. By this point, the cutch will have released its color and qualities to the lye, and you can strain out any remaining solid pieces as you add the solution to the oils and fats. Add 1 tablespoon (15 ml) of cutch per 5-pound (2.3-kg) batch of soap for warm reddish brown tones.

### ELDERBERRY (*Sambucus canadensis*)

**Nature:** This bushy shrub grows along the sides of the roads here in Tennessee — one of our most noticeable wildflowers, with its large feather-compound leaves, its large dill-like clusters of flowers, and, eventually, its dark purple berries. The cooked berries are edible and are also used as a violet fabric dye. The leaves are used as an emollient and to treat bruises and sprains. The leaves yield a yellow dye, but since the leaves, roots, and stems of some species are poisonous, I recommend avoiding these plant parts. The flowers are used in eye and skin lotions to soothe and soften, and in medicinal teas to treat colds. In large quantities, the flowers produce a soft yellow color in soaps; the berries, a pretty caramel color.

**Quantity/Procedure:** Add the flowers and/or berries to the fresh lye solution to steep for at least an hour. Per 5 pounds (2.3 kg) soap, use 1½ cups (375 ml) finely chopped fresh flowers, or 1½ cups (375 ml) crushed berries (or a combination of flowers and berries). Strain this lye solution before adding it to the fats and oils. The dark orange lye water fades in the final bars to light yellow (if you are using the flowers), or to caramel (if you are using the berries).

### GINSENG Chinese or Korean; American *(Panax ginseng; Panax quinquefolius)* Siberian *(Eleutherococus senticosus)*

**Nature:** The root of this plant is best known as an aphrodisiac because it is thought to stimulate male sex glands. But it is also used medicinally to strengthen the immune system, increase appetite, control blood pressure, and treat a variety of other conditions. It contains mucilage, resin, saponin, vitamins, and minerals.

Ginseng root grows best in a rich, virgin soil, and the quality of the root is dependent upon the quality of the soil. Only after five years in the ground are the roots ready to be harvested. The high cost of the finest ginseng is attributable to these demanding growing conditions. American ginseng is the most expensive today, because the supply from the wild has diminished and growing it organically is an expensive, long process. Chinese ginseng is grown commercially in less fertile soil and the final product is more affordable.

**Quantity/Procedure:** If I were choosing a ginseng root for medicinal purposes, I would choose the finer quality for the best effect. But since I believe that its medicinal properties are lost in the soapmaking process, I recommend choosing a less expensive ginseng root as a soap colorant. The Chinese ginseng root is the darkest in color; the others are lighter. Add the finely ground powder at the trace, just before adding scent to the soap. Ginseng contributes scent, color, and a fine texture to the final bars.

### GOLDENROD *(Solidago spp.)*

**Nature:** This prolific plant is considered a weed by some, but is one of my favorites. Its leaves and tall panicles of golden flowers yield a yellow dye. A contented goldenrod will spread out comfortably and produce year after year. Goldenrod produces astilbe-like flower heads with gold-yellow blossoms. These are used medicinally as a diuretic and to treat hay fever.

**Quantity/Procedure:** Lots of finely chopped, fresh goldenrod flowers (2¼ cups [550 ml] of flowers added to the lye solution per 5 pounds [2.3 kg] of soap) are required to achieve a most subtle yellow color in the soap. Use the flowers after they have opened but before they fade.

### GOLDENSEAL (Hydrastis canadensis)

**Nature:** This small perennial herb is somewhat controversial, with some claiming that it is one of the most important medicinal herbs, and others skeptical of its effectiveness and wary of its hydrastine content, thought to be toxic. Its thick, knotted, twisted yellow root stalk yields a yellow-orange dye. I'm unsure about using goldenseal as a soap colorant, so given the many yellows available, I recommend passing this one by.

Note: Because goldenseal is difficult to cultivate, it is gathered from the wild and can be scarce and expensive. Goldenseal was included as an official drug plant until 1936, when it came close to extinction due to overharvesting. Still today it is becoming endangered.

### HENNA (Lawsonia inermis)

**Nature:** Sometimes called red henna, the powdered leaves of this tropical perennial shrub produce a reddish yellow dye that is best known as a hair colorant. The lawsone found in the leaves is responsible for the orange color.

**Quantity/Procedure:** Add 1 tablespoon (15 ml) ground henna into the lye of a 5-pound (2.3-kg) batch for a sage green–brown color. Strain before adding to the fats and oils.

### LICORICE ROOT (Glycyrrhiza glabra)

**Nature:** The root of this shrub was used by the ancient Egyptian, Chinese, and Greek peoples to treat hoarseness and heartburn, and in an ointment to heal wounds. Today, licorice root is used medicinally as a demulcent, an emollient, and an anti-inflammatory. It is also thought to help open skin pores. The roots and stolons contain ingredients thought to prevent coughing, to have antiseptic properties, and to act as expectorants. The glycyrrhizin content of licorice root contributes to the retention of salt and water, so people with heart problems and pregnant women should not take it internally. Licorice root is an allergen for some individuals.

**Quantity/Procedure:**  The yellow coloring constituent found in the outer bark of the root adds an earthy yellow shade to a cold-process soap. Small pieces of the root (about ½ cup [125 ml] licorice root per 5 pounds [2.3 kg] soap) can be added to the freshly made lye solution and left to release its muddy yellow color for an hour or two. Strain out the root before adding the lye to the fats and oils. A full trace may be slightly delayed, as the mucilaginous parts of the root alter the consistency of the soap mixture somewhat.

### LOGWOOD *(Haematoxylon campechianum)*

**Nature:**  Logwood is obtained from a tree common to the West Indies and Central America, and contains haematoxylin (its coloring constituent). The interior of the living wood is yellow, but once exposed to air it changes to dark brown. Logwood is used to dye fabric red, but to prepare the wood for use as a dye, it is chipped and fermented and no longer safe to use medicinally. Untreated, the wood has been used as an astringent, though it is known to cause allergic reactions in sensitive individuals.

**Quantity/Procedure:**  Adding 2 tablespoons (30 ml) ground logwood to the lye solution (strain before use) produces a brick-brown color in soap. However, I do not recommend the use of logwood in a skin-care product.

### MADDER ROOT *(Rubia tinctorum)*

**Nature:**  Madder root is used as a dye and by the pharmaceutical industry to produce drugs. At first glance, this perennial does not seem noteworthy, with its prickly stems and leaves, and its flowers of less than ⅒ inch (.25 cm) in diameter. But from below the ground, its root calls for attention and gets plenty of it — both positive and negative. The root of the madder plant contains anthraquinones, chemical compounds that are used medicinally in small quantities, but in excess are carcinogenic.

There are around thirty-five varieties of the madder plant, but the thick, fleshy, reddish brown root of *Rubia tinctorum,* known as dyer's root, produces the best red dye. Alizarin is the pigment found in madder

## THE MATTER OF MADDER

Many of the important dyes are compounds called anthraquinones, including alizarin, the yellow and red pigment found in madder root. There are about fifty different kinds of anthraquinones, all slight variations of one another and of their parent compound — quinone. Some are used as dyes, others by the pharmaceutical industry to produce drugs. Alizarin in madder root consists of ruberythric acid, one of the anthraquinone glucosides (compounds of alcohol and glucose). Anthraquinones are found in aloe, madder, rhubarb, yellow dock, castor oil, senna, cascara, and buckthorn. They are also found in fungi, lichens, and insects. Carminic acid, the purplish red dyeing constituent in the cochineal beetle, is another natural anthraquinone.

Madder root was used medicinally in ancient Egypt, Persia, and India, and is still used today for its curative properties. It is used to treat wounds and as an astringent, a purgative, and a laxative. Anthraquinones from madder root and aloe vera are used medicinally to prevent the formation of kidney stones and reduce the size of existing stones. They are thought to bind calcium in the urinary tract and slow the growth of urinary calcium crystals. Doses of madder root and other anthraquinone plants must be carefully controlled to avoid griping and irritation.

### What's the Madder?

Today, there is much controversy concerning the safety of anthraquinones, including the alizarin in madder root. Research has found anthraquinones to be carcinogenic in certain concentrations but medicinally beneficial in controlled doses. Unfortunately for the soapmaker, none of the definitive research involves the infinitesimal amounts of anthraquinones found in diluted compounds in a final bar of soap colored with madder root. Many studies have proven the carcinogenic effect of anthraquinones in mice, but the line between beneficial and unsafe use has not yet been drawn. Low doses of anthraquinones are used to treat cancer; high doses cause cancer. Laypeople are left to exercise caution as we wait for more specific advice. In the end, it is likely that madder root — like so many other plants and their essential oils — has both helpful and harmful properties. Moderation allows us to use plants safely and beneficially, but excess leads to dangerous risk.

root. A derivative of alizarin is produced by oxidizing anthracene, a compound present in coal tar. Today, both madder root and anthracene have been replaced as dyes by the synthetic form of alizarin.

**Quantity/Procedure:** If you are comfortable using madder root, purchase it cut and sifted; then powder the coarse pieces in a coffee grinder. The powdered root releases the most color. Add it to the lye solution, and strain the lye before pouring it into the fats and oils. Approximately 1½ tablespoons (22.5 ml) finely ground madder root per 5 pounds (2.3 kg) soap will yield an antique pink-red color.

### MIMOSA (Albizia julibrissin)

**Nature:** The mimosa plant, also known as flowering acacia, which is naturalized in some parts of the South, offers shades of peach and tan to soap. This fast-growing tree has large fernlike leaves and beautiful pink and yellow silklike flowers with a wonderful scent.

**Quantity/Procedure:** I use large quantities of the leaves (strip the individual stems downward for quick removal of the small leaflets) to achieve a warm brown shade. Grind the leaves as finely as possible in a coffee grinder and use 1½ cups (375 ml) of the ground leaves per 5 pounds (2.3 kg) of soap. Add the plant material to the lye solution and let it steep for an hour or so, stirring occasionally to release more color. Strain the lye and add it to the fats and oils. The soap mixture eventually turns from a brown-brick color to mauve and, eventually, warm peachy tan.

### PAPRIKA (Capsicum annum)

**Nature:** Paprika is the deep red powder you buy in the grocery store spice section. It comes from the ground, dried fruits of this mild pepper.

**Quantity/Procedure:** Add ½–1 teaspoon (2–5 ml) paprika per pound of soap at the end of the process, just before pouring into molds. It produces a peach tint with russet specks. Too much paprika can be abrasive.

### QUEEN ANNE'S LACE (Daucus carota)

**Nature:** This vigorous biennial has stiff stems and broad, flat, white-green flower heads above stiff stems. It grows along the roads in some regions and self-seeds readily.

**Quantity/Procedure:** The entire plant yields shades of yellow in the dyepot. Steep the plant material in the lye solution (2 cups [500 ml] of Queen Anne's lace per 5 pounds [2.3 kg] of soap). Strain before adding the lye to the fats and oils.

### ROSE HIPS *(Rosa canina, Rosa arvensis, Rosa rubiginosa)*

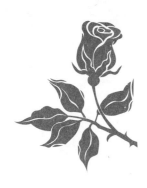

**Nature:** Roses produce berrylike fruit, known as rose hips, to hold the seeds. Once the flower has been fertilized, it drops its petals and the fruit (the rose hip) plumps and turns a beautiful shade of orange, pink, or scarlet. The rose hips from a variety of wild roses are used in medicines, teas, and preserves. Fresh rose hips contain more than twice as much vitamin C as fresh oranges. As a soap colorant, the most common rose hip powder available is derived from the species *Rosa canina.* Note that the seeds inside the hip of the species *Rosa rubiginosa* contain an oil, rosa mosqueta rose hip seed oil, that is high in essential fatty acids and is thought to speed the healing of skin lesions.

**Quantity/Procedure:** Cut and sifted rose hips can be ground into a beautiful rosy peach powder and added to soap just before you pour into molds. (I purchase the ground powder.) Use 2 tablespoons (30 ml) rose hip powder per 5 pounds (2.3 kg) soap for a pinkish tan color that is colorfast.

### SAFFLOWER *(Carthamus tincorius)*

**Nature:** Safflower is also known as false saffron, because the petals of its blossoms yield a diluted form of the yellow color of true saffron. Though it takes more than 4,000 dried saffron stigmas to produce an ounce (28 g) of dye, leaving saffron quite costly, very little dye is required to produce saffron's unique yellow color due to its principal pigment, crocin.

Safflower, with both yellow and red coloring matter, produces yellow, rose, and scarlet dyes, but much larger quantities are required to achieve even a diluted version of saffron. Safflower is an inexpensive alternative to saffron for the soapmaker looking for specks of fairly stable color in the final bars.

**Quantity/Procedure:** Because other colorants contribute more concentrated color using less plant material, these other yellow, red, and orange possibilities are better suited to complete coverage. I use safflower petals as threads of color and texture on a white background. Add approximately ½ cup (125 ml) safflower petals per 5 pounds (2.3 kg) soap at trace.

## SAFFRON *(Crocus sativus)*

**Nature:** The dried stigma of the saffron plant contains the glycoside crocin, a water-soluble yellow powder. There are only three stigmas in each flower, and 165,000 blossoms are required to make 1 kilogram (2.2 lbs.) of colorant, so the cost of saffron is high. Safflower can be substituted, but it is a weaker colorant.

## SAINT-JOHN'S-WORT *(Hypericum perforatum)*

**Nature:** One of my favorite plants in the garden, this hardy, fragrant perennial grows larger each year, producing hundreds of beautiful yellow, lemon-scented flowers. The red pigment in the flowers is called hypericin. The entire plant is used medicinally, especially as an astringent and to heal wounds. Saint-John's-wort oil is used to treat cuts and burns and as an astringent.

**Quantity/Procedure:** Harvest Saint-John's-wort flowers once they are fully opened for the deepest color. They yield a yellow dye in oil, alcohol, or lye. Per 5 pounds (2.3 kg) of soap, add ¼–½ cup (60–125 ml) of finely chopped fresh flowers to the freshly made lye solution and strain before using.

## SEAWEED

**Nature:** Thousands of species of seaweed meet the nutritional requirements of water animals in ponds, lakes, rivers, and oceans. Human skin and plant "skin" contain 90 percent water, and have pores to breathe and transmit nutrients, a protective layer to control moisture loss, and a mechanism to allow evaporation and cooling. The shared structures account for the resemblance of blood serum to seawater (they are chemically similar). Many of the nutrients people need to survive are found in the sea plants that keep water animals alive: vitamins A, B-complex, C, D, E, F, and K, iodine, magnesium, copper, zinc, iron, calcium, phosphorus, nitrogen, and manganese. Seaweed is richer in vitamins and minerals than land plants, and contains almost as much chlorophyll as alfalfa.

*Kelp.* Also known as bladderwrack *(Fucus vesiculosus),* kelp is one of the many algae. It is used medicinally because of its high concentration of silicon, vitamins, and calcium, but again, how effective these nutrients are in a cold-process soap is unclear. Kelp is considered a soothing, moisturizing plant and is used in mineral baths. Powdered kelp is soft and light, and it gently tints soap a very pale shade of gray-green.

*Dulse.* Another kind of seaweed, dulse *(Palmaria palmata)* is part of the red algae group that includes Irish moss as well as plants that contain agar-agar, the vegetarian substitute for gelatin. The mucilage in agar-agar helps to emulsify lotions and creams, and its gel feels soothing and soft. It is the agar-agar content that makes both Irish moss and dulse emollient. Dulse is darker than kelp and lighter than spirulina. Due to fading, it, too, contributes more texture than color to the final bars.

*Spirulina.* This blue-green algae contains a very high concentration of nutrients and is included in the diet to help absorb minerals and strengthen the immune system, since it is easily assimilated by the body. This particular alga is used to treat a wide range of health problems, including skin disorders. With its deep blue-green color, even after fading, spirulina is a lovely addition to any soap. Add ⅛–½ cup (30–125 ml) powdered spirulina per 5 pounds (2.3 kg) soap at the trace.

*Nori.* This seaweed *(Porphyra)* has a protein content of 40 percent and contains vitamins A, B-complex, and C. Compressed sheets of nori are used to make sushi rolls. Crush the sheets into coarse pieces or powder for green specks of color in your final bars. Add nori at the trace.

**Quantity/Procedure:** Though it is doubtful that seaweed retains its nutritive value after battling the lye, and though the colors fade in heat and light, coarse or powdered seaweed flakes contribute texture and subtle specks of color to your final bars.

### SOAPWORT *(Saponaria officinalis)*

**Nature:** Soapwort, also known as bouncing bet and latherwort, has been used since ancient time as a gentle cleanser. The saponin found in its roots and leaves is responsible for the sudsy lather produced when the plant parts are bruised and mixed with water. The soapy mixture is thought to relieve itching from eczema and other irritating skin conditions. Though some herbalists use soapwort tea medicinally, the internal use of soapwort is discouraged since saponin can be toxic. Soap colored with soapwort turns a beautiful, bright lime green, but after a week into the cure period, the soap fades to a muddier green/ yellow earth tone.

**Quantity/Procedure:** Add ½ tablespoon (7.5 ml) powdered soapwort leaf to the hot lye solution. Stir the lye occasionally to release more color and strain the leaves before adding the lye to the fats and oils.

### SUMAC BERRIES *(Rhus glabra* — dwarf sumac; *Rhus typhina* — staghorn sumac; *Rhus copallina* — smooth sumac)*

**Nature:** There are many varieties of sumac, a few of them poisonous, but the three listed above are nontoxic and produce dense clusters of small, dry, hairy red fruits at the ends of the branches. When ripe, the hard berries are covered with acidic red hairs.

**Quantity/Procedure:** Dry the berries, then grind them into a powder and add to the lye for a light, caramel brown color (4 tablespoons [60 ml] per 5 pounds [2.3 kg] soap). In more alkaline soap mixtures, the color will be more of an antique pink.

### TANSY *(Tanacetum vulgare)*

**Nature:** This perennial is known for its lush, fernlike leaves — which were strewn across the floors in English homes during the sixteenth and seventeenth centuries. Along with sweet Annie and Powis Castle, tansy is one of my favorite wreath-making herbs because of its unusual scent. Though tansy is also used medicinally, caution must be exercised. When used sparingly, tansy is effective, but in excess it can cause death. The dangerous constituent is thujone, and some varieties of tansy contain more thujone than others. Tansy is used in skin-care preparations, such as tonics and lotions, for its cleansing, soothing qualities. It is also used to treat acne.

**Quantity/Procedure:** Though tansy can be used as a soap colorant to achieve shades of green, I recommend choosing safer alternatives.

**CAUTION**

Do not use poison sumac, *Rhus vernix,* a small tree or shrub with hairless twigs and buds and 6–12 inch (15.25–30.5 cm) leafheads that have seven to thirteen pointed, toothless leaflets. The bark is smooth and speckled with black spots. This sumac has clusters of white berries, not red, and is often found in wooded swamps.

### TURMERIC *(Curcuma longa)*

**Nature:** The bulbous roots of this tender perennial have fragrant, dark orange flesh and can be ground into turmeric powder. Some turmeric powders are more yellow, others more orange. Turmeric root contains the anthraquinone 2-hydroxy-methyl-anthraquinone (see "Madder Root").

**Quantity/Procedure:** Add turmeric powder to the lye solution (about 1 teaspoon [5 ml] per cup [250 ml] of water) or to the final soap mixture just before you pour into a mold. The soap takes on shades of peach or orange. An added sprinkling of paprika is a nice touch.

### WALNUT HULLS AND LEAVES *(Juglans regia* — Persian walnut; *Juglans nigra* — American black walnut*)*

**Nature:** There are many varieties of walnut trees, including many edible fruit trees, timber trees, and ornamental trees. Two of the best-known species are Persian walnut and American black walnut; both are valued for their fine wood and quality nuts. The juice of the green husks, boiled with honey, is used medicinally to treat a sore mouth, an inflamed throat, and wounds. The walnut is used to treat eczema and other skin diseases. Tinctures made with the leaves and bark are used as astringents.

**Quantity/Procedure:** The green husks, also known as the hulls (the fresh outer covering), and shells of the Persian walnut fruit produce yellows and browns. The leaves of the American black walnut tree yield a brown dye; they are thought to contain iodine. I have not experimented with the leaves, but I add ¼ cup (60 ml) powdered walnut hulls per 5 pounds (2.3 kg) soap at the trace.

### WHEAT GERM *(Triticum aestivum)*

**Nature:** A part of the grass family, wheat is easy to grow. The wheat kernel consists of the germ, the bran, and the endosperm; the germ is the portion of the kernel from which the plant grows once the seed is sown. It is highly nutritious.

**Quantity/Procedure:** Wheat germ, isolated from the rest of the wheat berry, can be used for texture and color in soap. It can be included in any scrub soap for its scratch appeal, but be aware that it becomes

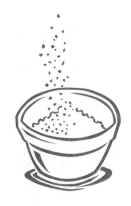

rancid rapidly. You can buy unprocessed wheat germ for the freshest material, though toasted wheat germ is fine and lasts longer. When wheat germ oil is used as a soapmaking oil and nutrient (from 10 to 30 percent of the total fats and oils), it lends a beautiful yellow-orange color to the final bars of soap, somewhat like one of the shades that annatto seed provides.

### DYER'S WOAD (*Isatis tinctoria*)

**Nature:** A blue paste from the fermented leaves of this biennial was used for 2,000 years in war paint, as well as medicinally, as an astringent and to control bleeding wounds. Because woad is considered toxic and unsafe to use internally, I recommend avoiding its external application as well.

### YARROW (*Achillea* spp.)

**Nature:** This perennial herb has large umbrel clusters of flowers that look like dill heads. Yarrow has been used medicinally to treat a wide range of symptoms, most commonly for wounds. It is thought to be a stimulant, an antispasmodic, and an anti-inflammatory. Yarrow contains a salicylic acid derivative (related to aspirin) that is thought to affect colds accompanied by fever. As a skin-care contribution, yarrow is astringent and cleansing; it is often found in natural creams and lotions.

**Quantity/Procedure:** The leaves and flower heads of nearly all of the different-colored yarrows yield a yellow-gold dye.

## OTHER MISCELLANEOUS COLORANTS

### CARAMEL

**Nature:** The caramel used as a colorant is nothing like the candy cubes melted to make caramel apples. Neither is it particularly natural anymore. Caramel coloring has been approved by the FDA for use in cosmetics. To make this colorant, sugar or glucose is heated with an alkali or a trace mineral acid, producing a burnt sugar. It can also be made from corn syrup by heating the syrup in the presence of catalysts to 250°F (121°C) for several hours, then cooling the mixture to 200°F (93°C). The brown color can come from true caramelization or from oxidative reactions. A good old-fashioned caramel powder can be made from sugar and water, to impart warm brown shades.

**Quantity/Procedure:** Combine 1 cup of sugar, ⅓ cup of water, and ⅛ teaspoon cream of tartar in a small heavy-bottomed saucepan and heat on medium (setting 6 or 7) until the sugar dissolves, whisking continuously. Increase heat to medium-high (setting 9); boil until mixture reaches 360°F (182°C). Set pan in bowl of cold water and quick-cool the caramel to 250°F (122°C). Spoon the caramel onto a triple layer of aluminum foil and cool completely before peeling away the foil. When room temperature, break caramel into pieces and grind into a powder using a food processor or coffee grinder. Store in tightly sealed container. (Soak sticky pans and utensils in very hot water to melt away caramel.)

Add 2–4 tablespoons of powdered caramel to the freshly made lye solution, stirring thoroughly to blend well. Stir periodically during the cool-down period to dissolve any small remaining pieces of caramel. Strain lye solution well before adding to fats and oils.

### OILS (FATTY AND VOLATILE)

Many soapmaking ingredients included for their nutritional contributions also lend color to the final soap. Consider including a meaningful percentage of the following nutrients to better utilize their offerings:

- Wheat germ oil (yellow-orange)
- Carrot root and carrot seed essential oil (yellow-orange)
- Unrefined palm oil (yellow-orange)
- Pomace olive oil (off-white to olive green, depending upon the harvest)
- Hemp seed oil, lower-grade (olive green)
- Cassia bark essential oil (yellow)
- Vanilla absolute (brown)

### RESINS (OLEORESINS, BALSAMS, AND GUMS)

**Nature:** Resins join the select group of colorants that contribute more than just color to soap. Most lend rich brown tones to the final bars, but they are also thought to affect a soap's skin-care value. Though resins can be sensitizers for some people, they have been used medicinally for thousands of years. A few also contribute a full-bodied, long-lasting scent.

**Quantity/Procedure:** Benzoin, tolu balsam, and Peru balsam are all dark brown liquid resins with heavy, lingering scents of vanilla. They darken all soaps to some shade of brown, depending upon the fats and oils in the formula and the amount of resin used. Dissolve the desired amount of resin in as little alcohol as possible to avoid seizing the soap. Add the resin/alcohol mixture with the essential oils at the trace. Resins are difficult to incorporate into cold-process soap in the large quantities most people want. See chapter 10, pages 206–207, for a fuller discussion.

### ULTRAMARINES

**Nature:** Ultramarine is no longer derived from the gem lapis lazuli. Instead, ultramarine pigments are made synthetically by heating a mixture of kaolin, sodium carbonate, sulfur, silica, carbon, and resin to very high temperatures. Ultramarine blue, pink, and violet share almost identical chemical formulas (see chapter 11, page 216).

**Quantity/Procedure:** Ultramarine is a synthetic colorant from beginning to end. There's nothing natural about it, and yet I am not aware of any studies that have found synthetic ultramarines toxic or sensitizing. The FDA has approved this colorant, claiming that it is nontoxic and inert, and though I have some concerns and remain alert to new findings, many soapmakers seem to be using ultramarines safely, including me. Using them in moderation makes good sense, however, since many synthetic colorants that at first seem inert, later prove to be irritating. Fortunately, only 1 teaspoon (5 ml) of ultramarine is needed to color 5 pounds (2.3 kg) of soap spectacular shades of blue. This product is insoluble in water, but can be incorporated into raw soap before it is poured into molds, or into the lye solution (cooled to 80 to 100°F) for best incorporation. When adding it to the soap, add ultramarine immediately after adding the lye solution to the fats and oils. Force the powder through the finest mesh tea strainer to avoid unblended particles in the final bars of soap.

---

## COLORS OBTAINED FROM ULTRAMARINES

**Ultramarine Blue**
◆ Dark, sapphire blue:
1½–2 teaspoons (7–10 ml) per 5 pounds (2.3 kg) soap
◆ Robin's-egg blue:
½ teaspoon (2 ml) per 5 pounds (2.3 kg) of soap;
◆ Light blue:
¼ teaspoon (1 ml) per 5 pounds (2.3 kg) soap

**Ultramarine Rose**
◆ Bright pink:
4 teaspoons (20 ml) per 5 pounds (2.3 kg) soap
◆ Mauve:
Use ½ part milk, ½ part water for the lye solution; add ½ tablespoon (7.5 ml) ultramarine rose per 5 pounds (2.3 kg) soap (the pink is prettiest within a milk soap, where it turns a darker shade of mauve instead of a candy pink)

**Ultramarine Violet**
◆ Beautiful purple-violet:
3 teaspoons (45 ml) per 5 pounds (2.3 kg) soap (less for lighter shades of lavender)

### CLAYS AND MINERALS

**Nature:** See chapter 11 for more details about iron oxides, kaolin, montmorillonite, ultramarines, titanium dioxide, ochers, pearlescent pigments, and red hematite.

**Quantity/Procedure:** All of these substances contribute color to soap as their fine particles are dispersed evenly throughout the mixture. They do not combine chemically with the other soapmaking ingredients and are usually added at the trace, before the essential oil. Ochers usually lend brown and yellow shades to soap; red iron oxide lends various shades of bluish red and yellowish red. Montmorillonite (also known as bentonite or French green clay) is a subtle gray-green and is used by some soapmakers for a hint of color. Some companies sell a red clay that is described as montmorillonite, but real montmorillonite is not red. Most of this "red clay" is actually a mixture of montmorillonite and synthetic red iron oxide. Titanium dioxide whitens the soap and can be added to the marbled portion of the batch for white-on-white (bright white swirls against an off-white background). It is also used as a blending color, to create lighter shades of the darker minerals. When red iron oxide is combined with titanium dioxide, a rosy pink color is achieved.

## CAUTION

The FDA has approved synthetic iron oxide, titanium dioxide, ultramarines, and other iron oxides as safe cosmetic colorants, but FDA approval is no guarantee of safety. Note that many once-approved coal-tar dyes have been dropped from the FDA's approved list one by one. The marketplace is full of adulterated versions of these colorants, with no affordable check-and-balance system. You, the soapmaker, must rely on material safety data sheets completed by the supplier (see chapter 13, page 248) — unless a laboratory and chemist happen into your life.

I recommend some careful consideration before using these materials in a skin-care product. Once again, maybe they're harmless and maybe they're not. Most chemists give full endorsements, and only a few seem concerned. But those who are concerned raise questions of purity and allergic reactions and some chronic conditions, so I've decided that the upside (one of many color opportunities) is not worth the potential downside. If you are comfortable using these colorants, do your best to distinguish the higher grades from the lower ones. Periodically pay a laboratory to test a small sample for impurities.

# CHAPTER 6
## Creating Scents from Around the World

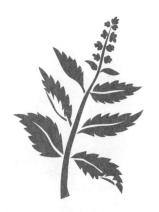

Dr. Louis Leakey, the late anthropologist, believed that early humans survived for millions of years because predators were repulsed by their scent and often let them be. He suggested that this natural defense protected people before they had learned to design weapons, and that as weapons became more prevalent, body odor diminished. Today's body odors are pretty tame, though some would dispute this claim.

Not only were primitive people able to repel by odor, their sense of smell was also more acute than ours. Prehistoric warriors could smell predators from great distances. Since the ability to provide and defend depended upon a good sense of smell, it was a matter of survival.

People today can distinguish one scent from another to only a limited degree, and many are easily misled. Others have lost their sense of smell entirely and get along fine. The sense of smell only helps us modern-day people survive in most unusual circumstances. Odor may kill a social life, but it no longer determines biological life and death.

## Necessity to Narcissism

Still, the sense of smell is not irrelevant to our lives. The success of the perfume industry tells us this. That people will pay inflated prices for special and not-so-special blends suggests that we value scent even if we don't need it. Scent may still help us attract mates, though I suspect that more people are attracted to someone's natural scent than to the latest bottle of masculine musk or femme fatale.

Today we get more pleasure than protection from fragrance: We drink in the scent of blossoms, light scented candles, burn incense, spray rooms with scent, and have successfully pushed industry to scent every product imaginable.

Yes, we are still people aware of scent, and acutely aware of appearance and presentation. Rather than applying a light touch of a favorite scent, we often drench ourselves in it to be sure that there's plenty. And there is! We go to extremes to avoid body odor, even accepting rashes from synthetic deodorants rather than go without. Some countries are more tolerant of natural odors than others; in my life, the only day without deodorant is a day spent alone.

## SCENT AND THE PSYCHE

Humans and animals like and dislike certain scents. Some people love to smell gasoline fumes as they pump gas into their cars; many horse lovers enjoy the smell of the stalls; photographers seem immune to the scent of their developing chemicals; some parts of the world love the smell of rancid fat. On the other hand, the smells of isopropyl alcohol and germicides cause tension by invoking memories of past visits to the doctor. Even our pets put on the brakes as they enter the veterinarian's office, and I don't think they're relying only upon memory.

We know that people can be so affected by scent that they associate good and bad scents with good and bad memories. Even offensive smells can become fond memories when associated with a good happening. And, conversely, normally intoxicating scents can remind us of bad times when associated with unhappy occasions. The effect of a scent on our psyches depends upon its associations. The lasting impressions of my times in Maine are associated with the smell of the pine trees. It is probably not a coincidence that we have chosen a home here in Tennessee surrounded by southern loblolly pines.

## "You Can't Argue with Taste"

Scents are more and less popular in different parts of the world. Patchouli or ylang-ylang may be considered heady and sensual in one area, and nauseating in another. Both the medicinal and the emotional powers of essential oils have been long recognized, even the self-induced power of imagined effect. Women in the Near East once provided their mates with handkerchiefs to tuck into their armpits through a hot day of manual labor. These women delighted in the smell of body odor. I've been spoiled by showers and soap and cologne, and cannot appreciate this aphrodisiac.

## SCENT IN SOAP

I devote as much attention to scenting my soap as I do to ensuring its effectiveness. In a day when many of us are fortunate enough to derive some leisure and pleasure from bathing, fragrance is an important soap trait, just as lather and hardness are. After devoting much time, expense, and attention to the soapmaking process, don't be indifferent to the final step of scenting the soap — unless, of course, you prefer unscented soap. Mediocre or off blends can spoil an otherwise wonderful batch of soap.

Half of the fun of soapmaking is experimenting with different blends of essential oils. Enjoy your creative license and mix and match in small quantities. Keep a good reference book nearby and feel comfortable substituting a related essential oil for one that is exorbitantly expensive. One piece of good news: You can add much less scent when using the finest-quality pure essential oils. The cheaper adulterated oils don't go so far.

### Regional Blends

Particular scents are often connected with certain parts of the world, because the plants from which the scents are derived are native to those regions and intimately associated with them. Countries that are blessed with a raw material to export often explore its potential, exploiting any and all uses for it. Regions are in some ways defined by these resources and their by-products.

The following list includes a few of the more popular blends of essential oils in each of thirty different regions, ranging from just one blend in several regions to as many as fifteen blends in France. I've also included my own favorites. As you blend the essential oils, always test their ratios in small quantities, and feel free to add extra scents or substitute others.

**BEWARE THE POWER OF SCENT**

In eighteenth-century England, certain scents were sold as magic potions. Salesmen claimed that they would make all women more beautiful. Parliament passed a law during the reign of King George III in 1774 that revealingly stated:

"All women, of whatever age, rank, profession or degree whatever, virgins, maids or widows, that shall from and after this act impose upon, seduce and betray into matrimony any of His Majesty's subjects by the use of scents, paints, cosmetics, washes, artificial teeth, false hair, Spanish wool [a kind of rouge], iron stays, hoops, high-heeled shoes or bolstered hips, shall incur the penalty of the law now in force against witchcraft and like misdemeanors, and that the marriage, upon conviction, shall stand null and void."

The intoxicating nature of scents, real and imagined, was clearly understood.

## MY FAVORITE SCENT COMBINATIONS (TENNESSEE, USA)

*The amounts given for these essential oil blends are in measured teaspoons (1 teaspoon = approximately 5 ml). Each formula will scent 5 pounds (2.3 kg) of soap.*

Basil (1¼), Lime (2¼), Orange (2¼), Rosemary (1¼)

Bergamot (2), Lavender (3), Lemon (1), Lime (1)

Jasmine (2¾), Sweet orange (2¾), Vetiver (1½)

Lavender (1), Palmarosa (3), Sandalwood (3)

Bergamot (2), Caraway (1½), Cassia (1¼), Cloves (1½), Sassafras (¾)

Clary sage (2½), Lavender (¼), Rose geranium (3¼), Sandalwood (1)

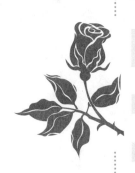

Bois de rose (1), Frangipani (¾), Patchouli (¼), Peru balsam (3), Sandalwood (1¼), Ylang-ylang (¾)

Cassia (½), Juniper berry (½), Rose (3), Sandalwood (3)

Almond (1), Bergamot (1¼), Cassia (1), Cloves (3¾)

Cloves (1¼), Lavender (¾), Patchouli (2), Ylang-ylang (3)

Juniper berry (2¼), Lavender (1½), Rosemary (1¼), Thyme (2)

Basil (1¼), Juniper berry (2½), Lemon (2¼), Patchouli (1)

Palmarosa (2¼), Patchouli (2¼), Sweet orange (2¼)

Cloves (1), Lime (1), Patchouli (1½), Sandalwood (3½)

Bay laurel (3), Clary sage (1), Juniper berry (1), Siberian fir needle (2)

Clove (2), Geranium (3), Juniper berry (1), Patchouli (1)

## Africa
- Cedarwood, lavender, marjoram, tea tree, thyme

## Antigua
- Bergamot, geranium, neroli, orange, rose attar, sandalwood, vanilla, violet
- Magnolia

## Antilles
- Lemon, lime

## Austria
- Cinnamon, lavender, lemon, peppermint, rosemary, sage

## Bulgaria
- Cassia (acacia), jasmine, orange, rose, violet

## Burma
- Frangipani, jasmine, sandalwood

## China and Japan
- Bergamot, caraway, cardamom, cloves, rose, sandalwood
- Jasmine, muguet, sandalwood
- Chamomile, frankincense, lavender, myrrh, oakmoss, rose, vanilla
- Black pepper, cinnamon, cloves, ginger, frankincense, nutmeg
- Cassia, cloves, geranium, palmarosa, patchouli
- Cinnamon, cloves, geranium, jasmine, lavender, patchouli, sandalwood, star anise, sweet orange, vanilla, vetiver, ylang-ylang
- Bergamot, caraway, cassia, cinnamon, cloves, geranium, lemon, nutmeg, orange, patchouli, tea tree
- Cardamom, cinnamon, cloves, coriander, geranium, jasmine, narcissus, orris root, patchouli, rose, ylang-ylang
- Allspice, ylang-ylang

### East Indies

- Jasmine, lavender, patchouli, vetiver, ylang-ylang
- Rose, vetiver

### El Salvador

- Heliotrope, Peru balsam, tolu balsam, vanilla

### England

- Violet, heather
- Cedarwood, jasmine, lavender, rosemary
- Cloves, mint, rose
- Geranium, lavender flower, patchouli, palmarosa, spike lavender
- Benzoin, cloves, juniper berry, lemon, rose

### France

- Jasmine, muguet, rose, sandalwood
- Basil, jonquil, violet
- Jasmine, petitgrain, rose, ylang-ylang
- Lavender, oakmoss
- Lily of the valley, rose
- Clary sage, violet
- Bergamot, clary sage, lavender, oakmoss
- Bergamot, patchouli, tolu balsam, vanilla, violet, ylang-ylang
- Cassia, cloves, orris root, rose, sandalwood
- Bergamot, clary sage, jasmine, labdanum, lemon, oakmoss, patchouli, rose
- Almond, bergamot, cloves, jasmine, orange, rose, tuberose, vanilla, violet
- Cardamom, jasmine, lily of the valley, orange, violet
- Rose, violet
- Narcissus, sandalwood, vetiver
- Jasmine, oakmoss, orange, tuberose

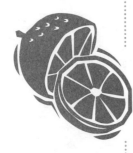

### French Guiana/Brazil

- Bois de rose, lilac, lily, mignonette, orange, rose

### Germany

- Bergamot, cinnamon, lavender, lemongrass, neroli, rose geranium, rosemary, sweet orange

### Greece
- Anise, cloves
- Anise, caraway, cloves
- Bay, citrus, patchouli, spice

### Holland
- Clary sage, nutmeg, oakmoss, Peru balsam

### India
- Clary sage, jasmine, oakmoss, patchouli, vetiver, violet, ylang-ylang
- Patchouli, rose, sandalwood

### Italy and Spain
- Calamus, coriander, jasmine, orris root, rose
- Lemon, orange

### Jamaica
- Allspice, geranium, lavender, patchouli, ylang-ylang
- White birch

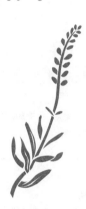

### Java and Sri Lanka
- Bergamot, citronella, geranium, pine

### Marquesas Islands
- Lavender, patchouli, Peru balsam, ylang-ylang
- Patchouli, Peru balsam, petitgrain, rose, sandalwood

### Philippine Islands
- Champaca magnolia, clary sage, sandalwood, violet
- Jasmine, Peru balsam, rosewood, vetiver, ylang-ylang

### Riviera
- Carnation, jasmine, marjoram, narcissus, tuberose, violet

### Scotland
- Carnation, cedarwood, jasmine, lilac, myrrh, orange blossom, sandalwood, ylang-ylang
- Bergamot, caraway, cassia, cloves, geranium

### South America
- Frangipani, ylang-ylang
- Narcissus, sandalwood, vetiver
- Jasmine, oakmoss, orange blossom, rose, violet
- Coriander, oakmoss, sassafras, vanilla, ylang-ylang
- Coumarin, musk, oakmoss, patchouli, vetiver
- Carnation, coreopsis, heliotrope, tuberose, violet

### Sri Lanka, Zanzibar, Sumatra, and India
- Cassia, cinnamon, cloves, orange, Peru balsam, ylang-ylang

### Tahiti
- Benzoin, frangipani, frankincense, jasmine, sandalwood

### Tanzania
- Dill, eucalyptus, rosemary

### Thailand/Indonesia
- Benzoin, coriander, frankincense, jasmine, juniper berry, lemon, myrrh, rose, sandalwood
- Frankincense, myrrh, rose, sandalwood

### United States of America
- Cedar, peppermint, sassafras, spearmint, wintergreen

### West Indies
- Cloves, orange, West Indian bay
- Allspice, patchouli, West Indian bay
- Allspice, geranium, lavender, rosemary, ylang-ylang

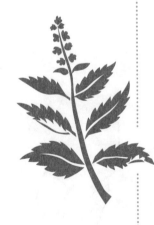

## CHAPTER 7
### Determining Soapmaking Temperatures

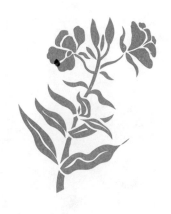

$S$oapmakers' preferences probably differ most with respect to the soapmaking temperatures. Some mix the lye and the fats and oils at about the same temperatures; some use high temperatures for the fats and oils and low temperatures for the lye solution; others go by feel and pour the lye into the fats and oils when both mixtures are no longer hot to the touch. When I first started making soap, I was slavishly attentive to temperature. But after using many combinations of temperatures, I have realized with relief and amazement that most of the soaps turned out fine. Though some formulas are better suited to particular temperatures, most soap can be made using a wide range. I've made it at 140°F (60°C), at 60°F (15.5°C), and at many temperatures in between. After comparing the processing temperature's effect on the chemical and physical characteristics of the saponifying soap mixture and the final bars, I've arrived at some personal preferences. But there is no one best soapmaking temperature. The extremes should be avoided, but that leaves a wide range of acceptable temperatures. The recipes in this book that require particular temperatures note this. Otherwise, you can assume that your favorite soapmaking temperatures will work just fine.

## THE EFFECTS OF TEMPERATURE

I make larger batches (12 or more pounds [5.4 or more kg]) of my highly unsaturated soap (the unsaturated oil in the formula accounts for at least 50 percent of the total fat and oils) at 80°F (27°C) when I apply a 10 to 15 percent sodium hydroxide discount. I produce highly saturated soap (formulas containing a high percentage of saturated fats and oils) and marbled soap at 95–100°F (35–38°C). The soaps I make at 100°F (38°C) and above are those that contain high percentages of beeswax or cocoa butter, formulas to which I apply a 0 to 9 percent sodium hydroxide discount, and, of course, transparent and liquid soaps. Even though soapmaking works at many temperatures, you should understand how integrally the temperature affects the process and, sometimes, the final product. I have observed at least the following effects.

## Tracing Time

Tracing time is a measure of how much sodium hydroxide reacts with the fats and oils per unit of time. It is directly related to the stirring speed, the degree of saturation of the fats and oils, the strength of the lye solution, the percentage of water used, and sometimes the soapmaking temperatures.

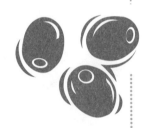

A brisk stir speeds up the reaction and a leisurely stir slows it down. Highly saturated formulas trace more quickly than do highly unsaturated ones. Stronger lye solutions cause quicker traces than do weaker solutions. And formulas that incorporate too much water are slower to trace. The lower temperatures (80–90°F, or 27–32°C) usually bring about the quickest traces for formulas with high percentages of unsaturated fats and oils (at least 50 percent of the total fats and oils), but when you're stirring quickly enough saturated formulas seem to trace quickly at any temperature between 80°F and 130°F (27°C and 54.5°C).

## Tolerance for Additives

Some nutrients and essential oils don't react as well or as reliably at extreme temperatures (below 75°F [23.8°C] and above 120°F [49°C]). Soap produced at these very low and very high temperatures is more likely to undergo chemical changes when exposed to room-temperature nutrients and essential and fragrance oils. Temperatures of 80–100°F (27–38°C) produce a soap mixture that better accepts these additives.

Most essential oils tolerate a wide range of soapmaking temperatures without seizing the soap, causing separation, or reversing the saponification process. Two exceptions are clove and cassia oil, both of which have trouble in warmer and colder batches. Synthetic fragrance oils can be troublesome at any temperature — though again, they better tolerate lower and midrange temperatures. Unfortunately, patterns cannot be drawn according to scent, since one company's gardenia or jasmine can be chemically different from another's. Test new scents on small soap batches, and add nutrients and scents at temperatures that minimize shock.

## Stability of Components

Often, the most valuable components in fats and oils (such as essential fatty acids) and nutrients (enzymes and vitamins) are also the least stable. They may not survive extended exposure to high temperatures. Such components are better preserved at lower soapmaking temperatures.

## Waiting Time

Some soapmakers love higher temperatures because they don't have to wait long to pour the lye into the fats and oils. Waiting for both mixtures to cool to 80°F (27°C) takes longer than waiting for them to reach a higher temperature. Should lower temperatures be your preference, remember that the cooling mixtures can be tucked aside and forgotten for a while while you attend to other matters. The lye solution can be prepared ahead of time in larger quantities and used at room temperature (65–80°F, or 18–27°C) along with the warmer fats and oils (110–120°F, or 43–49°C). Be sure to store the premixed lye solution in a perfectly sealed container; otherwise, the solution will weaken over time.

## Grain of Soaps

Most people don't notice any difference between the grains of soaps made at lower and those made at higher temperatures. I find that soaps made at the lower range have a dense, moist, fine grain — compared to the somewhat dryer, larger grain of soaps made at very high temperatures. The grain is also made smoother by superfatting with excess oils. This is an aesthetic issue only.

## Curdling in Bars

The higher the processing temperature, the more vulnerable the soap mixture is to curdling — the formation of solid, white, pearl-like pieces that remain in the final bars. Curdling is less likely to be a problem if you are using a mechanical mixer, since the stirring speed is fast and consistent. If you take even short breaks when hand-stirring, though, a hot soap mixture is likely to curdle. Just as a hot egg mixture can curdle when it's not whisked quickly enough, hot soap must be stirred quickly and consistently to avoid curdling. A curdled batch is a ruined batch, so be attentive to the speed of your stir when pushing soap to the higher soapmaking temperatures.

## Completing Saponification

Once soap has cured and is ready to use, all of the available lye should have reacted with all of the available fats and oils. Only a portion of the ingredients have united and reacted by the time the soap mixture is poured into molds; the remainder of the saponification reaction occurs during the insulation period and the cure.

The saponification reaction is heat-driven — it depends upon some heat for momentum. Though no external heat is applied to the soap mixture, the reaction itself produces heat that the soap retains and uses to keep the reaction going. The question is: How much heat is required to make soap? Warm temperatures certainly produce well-saponified bars of soap, but so do cooler ones. It's generally understood that warmer mixtures have better fluidity and solubility, and that higher processing temperatures allow soap ingredients more contact and more opportunity to react. Soap seems to both follow this rule and defy it. The superfatted soap I make at 80°F (27°C) traces, hardens, cures, and tests chemically much like the soap I make at higher temperatures. A soapmaker friend who takes no discount at all makes her fully saponified soap at 80–90°F (27–32°C). Final bars that she produces at 80°F (27°C) seem to be no less saponified than those produced at 140°F (60°)C — the reactants in both eventually combine, react, and produce good-quality soap. And though more of a hot soap mixture than of a cooler soap mixture has saponified by the time of the trace, this disparity is probably small when comparing soaps made at more common cold-process temperatures such as 80°F, 95°F, and 110°F (27°C, 35°C, and 43°C).

Even at the higher end of its temperature range, a cold-process soap has not completely saponified when it's ready to be poured into the mold; the remainder of the reaction takes place during the twenty-four-hour insulation period and the three-week cure. It is unclear how much of this reaction has taken place before pouring the soap, though figures of between 40 and 50 percent are the chemists' best estimates. It is pretty clear that batches produced at the higher temperatures (120–140°F, or 49–60°C) and stirred for longer periods of time probably contain more saponified soap at the time of pouring than soap made at cooler temperatures and stirred for only ten to fifteen minutes. But both warmer and cooler mixtures complete the reaction in the molds if the soap has been well blended into an emulsion, if the reactants are distributed evenly, and if the insulation temperatures aren't cold or hot.

## Ability to Try Special Techniques

Midrange temperatures produce a soap that is better able to wait for you while you make last-minute changes. The more extreme temperatures at either end continue on without you. Once a 130°F (54.4°C) batch or an 80°F (27°C) batch is close to tracing, neither can wait long for you to measure the essential oil you forgot to prepare ahead of time. And neither is well suited to marbling; the poured soap sets quickly, sometimes before the contrasting color has been thoroughly worked in. For batches that involve more craftsmanship, the midrange is best.

## Fluidity During Process

Soap made at midrange temperatures (95–105°F, or 35–41°C) develops greater fluidity during the soapmaking process, sometimes even after you've added scent and poured. Because the emulsion is less thick, separation in the mold is somewhat more of a risk with these temperatures,

### A RECOMMENDATION

Though even fully saponified soap made without taking a sodium hydroxide discount can be processed at 80°F (27°C), I don't recommend such low temperatures for small batches of fully saponified soap. Instead, I recommend a soapmaking temperature of 100°F (38°C), for better solubility. An experienced soapmaker can fully incorporate the extra percentage of sodium hydroxide even at the lower temperatures with a heavy-handed stir, but a few extra degrees of heat hedges the bet. I also urge those of you who take smaller sodium hydroxide discounts to use mechanical mixers; a conscientious hand-stir can do the job, but the mixer ensures a thorough saponification.

but it can be avoided by never pouring before achieving at least a light trace. When a formula incorporates many ingredients after the trace, a more fluid mixture allows you some time to add them without panicking. It doesn't seize and thicken as quickly as a batch made using higher or lower temperatures.

## Separation of Ingredients

Soap made at the lower temperatures rarely separates in the soapmaking pan or in the molds. I have never experienced separation using my 80°F (27°C) temperatures. Separation in the soapmaking pan results when the ingredients are not kept in motion, or when high temperatures precipitate certain ingredients out of solution. Separation in the molds results when soap produced at high temperatures cools too quickly; once under wraps, the hot soap cannot retain its high temperature and loses a certain amount of heat to the environment.

## Curdling in Molds

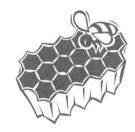

Soap made at high temperatures can be kept warmer under wraps by using the best insulators, but soap that retains too much heat in the molds can curdle in spots — usually in the center of the molds, where the temperatures are highest. Soap made using lower or midrange temperatures does not experience curdling in the molds. Again, watch for this potential result of using high temperatures. Never insulate more than two large trays (forty 5-ounce [141.75-g] bars per tray) together under the same wrap; too much heat is generated, and the innermost bars may curdle, either on their tops or their bottoms.

## Incorporating Ingredients with Higher Melting Points

Beeswax, an oil-soluble material with a high melting point, is best added with the other fats and oils so that it can saponify right along with them. If added at the trace, the melted beeswax solidifies into small pieces that will remain in the final bars. Lower processing temperatures do not interfere with the saponification of hydrogenated fats and oils that have melting points of between 76°F and 110°F (24.4°C and 43°C), but a material such as beeswax has a melting point close to 140°F (60°C) and requires higher processing temperatures.

## Ability to Produce Small Batches

Heat and stirring directly affect the saponification reaction, though not a tremendous amount of heat is required. Small batches retain less heat than larger batches and are usually produced at slightly higher soapmaking temperatures. Though the 80°F (27°C) temperatures generate enough heat to drive the saponification reaction to completion when stirring is brisk and continuous, I recommend producing small batches (less than 5 pounds, or 2.3 kg) of soap at processing temperatures of between 100°F and 110°F (38°C and 43°C).

## Summary

Before choosing your soapmaking temperatures, determine which soapmaking traits are most desirable to you, in order of preference, and then which temperatures achieve those traits. You may prefer the grain of the cooler- or warmer-processed soap. You may want a less temperamental mixture that is less likely to curdle. Your desired scents may be best incorporated within a certain range of temperatures. You may want to incorporate certain nutrients that lose essential components when exposed to high temperatures. Or you may prefer the convenience of not having to wait for oils and lye to cool down quite so long. No one temperature range will produce all of the desired traits, but you can determine which one satisfies more of your soapmaking needs.

# PROCESSING TEMPERATURES AND SOAPMAKING CHARACTERISTICS

| Soap Characteristic | 80–90°F (27–32°C) | 95–105°F (35–40.5°C) | 110–120°F (43–49°C) | 125–140°F (51.6–60°C) |
|---|---|---|---|---|
| Quick trace for batch of 5 pounds or less with quick hand-stirring | X | X | X | X |
| Quick trace for batch of more than 5 pounds with quick hand-stirring | X | X | X | X |
| Quick trace with quick mechanical mixing | X | X | X | X |
| More complete saponification upon pouring | | | X | X |
| Small batch (less than 5 pounds of soap) | | X | | |
| Finer-grained soap | X | X | | |
| Less reactive to scent (less likely to seize) | X | X | | |
| Less destructive to nutrients | X | X | | |
| Less vulnerable to curdling | X | X | | |
| More leisurely process (can make last-minute additions without rushing to avoid too thick a mixture) | | X | | |
| Shorter cool-down time for lye and fats/oils | | | X | X |
| Avoid hot spots | X | X | | |
| More fluid soap | | X | | |
| No separation | X | | | |
| Accommodates ingredients with higher melting points | | | X | X |

# CHAPTER 8
## Diagnosing Signs of Trouble

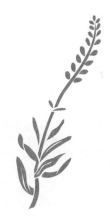

Early in my soapmaking days, another soapmaker encouraged me to take careful notes of each and every soapmaking. I was told to record the exact amounts of the ingredients used, along with a detailed discussion of the process from beginning to end. Benefiting from my many failed batches, you should experience very few of the following pitfalls, but careful note-taking will help you avoid making the same mistakes twice.

Nearly all of the problems I've listed in this chapter are related to imprecision. To avoid the majority of them, follow the directions carefully and regularly test your scales and thermometers for accuracy. Remember, as frustrating as you'll find the occasional failure, most mistakes are small, and soap is forgiving. The major goofs are lifetime lessons.

## DIAGNOSING SIGNS OF TROUBLE WITHIN THE SOAP PAN

| Trouble Sign | Reasons Why | What to Do |
|---|---|---|
| Mixture in pan not tracing | ◆ Not enough lye<br>◆ Too much water<br>◆ Incorrect temperatures<br>◆ Stirring too slowly | Check your measurements to be sure that the correct amounts were used; check that your temperatures are within the recommended range; be sure that you are stirring briskly and consistently. If everything seems to be on track, continue stirring for as long as you can manage, but no longer than four hours. If the mixture separates into oily and watery layers, even after a few hours, give up on the batch. If in time it does begin to thicken meaningfully, go ahead and pour the nearly saponified batch, and allow the soap a normal cure period. Hope for the best, but be prepared for unusable soap.<br><br>Some superfatted vegetable soap formulas, made with high percentages of unsaturated oils, with no more than 20 percent |

*(continued on next page)*

| Trouble Sign | Reasons Why | What to Do |
|---|---|---|
| Mixture in pan not tracing (continued) | | coconut oil, with a minimum requirement of sodium hydroxide, and without palm oil or tallow, can be made over a ten to sixteen hour period, using a casual stir method. But the recipes in this book are formulated to saponify within seven to sixty minutes; hours and hours of processing would signal a problem. |
| Curdled mixture (small, pearly pebbles forming near the bottom of the pan) | ◆ Oils, lye, or both poured at too high a temperature<br>◆ Irregular stirring<br>◆ Stirring process was too slow | Pour the soap mixture once it has saponified, but if the final soaps are filled with these irregularities (and they probably will be), do not use the final bars. |
| Slightly grainy mixture | ◆ Soap was made using temperatures which were very high or very low<br>◆ Stirring process was not brisk and constant | This is an aesthetic problem only. |
| Mixture in pan beginning to set up prematurely (seizing) | ◆ Temperatures used were too high or too low<br>◆ Fats/oils are overreacting to synthetic fragrance<br>◆ Fats/oils are overreacting to certain pure essential oils, like clove or cassia<br>◆ Too high a percentage of saturated fats in formula | Carefully, but quickly, pour soap mixture into the frames, using a spatula to scoop out the firmer soap. Do your best to level the soap in the frame, as you would spread cake batter toward the edges of a cakepan. Proceed as usual. |
| Mixture in pan suddenly begins to streak | ◆ Synthetic fragrance oils made with alcohol or dipropylene glycol were used to scent the soap<br>◆ Soapmaking temperatures were too cold | If the mixture seems otherwise correct, and it has saponified, quickly pour the soap mixture into the frame. This is an aesthetic problem only, with what you might even consider to be an interesting design within the final bars. |

## DIAGNOSING SIGNS OF TROUBLE IN THE FINAL SOAPS

| Trouble Sign | Reasons Why | What to Do |
|---|---|---|
| Soaps marbled with white streaks (a swirled design; not solid white pieces) | ◆ Uneven emulsion from uneven stirring<br>◆ Temperatures of oils and lye too cold<br>◆ Synthetic fragrance oils used to scent the soap<br>◆ Stirred too long after adding fragrance | Be sure that these white swirls are not shiny, alkaline chunks of lye. Swirls created by the fragrance do not affect the purity of the soap. |
| Soft, spongy soap | ◆ Not enough sodium hydroxide<br>◆ Too much water | You can try to cure these for a longer period (a few more weeks), but it is unlikely that these will become firm enough for bar soap. |
| Hard, brittle soap | ◆ Too much sodium hydroxide | Do not use these bars. They are probably quite alkaline, with a significant excess of sodium hydroxide. |
| Cosmetic air bubbles | ◆ Stirred too long (soap should have been poured into the frames sooner)<br>◆ Stirred too quickly, more like whipping or beating | Be sure that these holes are not filled with lye. If they are just air bubbles, the soaps are fine. |
| Separation — greasy layer (unsaponified oils) on top of hard soap (harsh soap with excess lye) | ◆ Insufficient stirring<br>◆ Inaccurate proportion of fats/oils to sodium hydroxide (too much sodium hydroxide)<br>◆ Too quick a temperature drop in the frames<br>◆ Soap poured into frames too soon | Do not use these. Parts of these bars will be highly alkaline. Consider these unsafe for personal use. |
| Hard soap with bright white areas (not streaks, but random chunks of slippery solid lye) | ◆ Too much sodium hydroxide used<br>◆ Stirring process was too slow or inconsistent<br>◆ Too much sodium hydroxide | Do not use these bars — the chunks of lye will burn.<br><br>*(continued on next page)* |

| Trouble Sign | Reasons Why | What to Do |
|---|---|---|
| Excessive amount of white powder on top of bars, or cakey, crumbly slab of soap | ◆ Hard water used to dissolve the sodium hydroxide | Do not use these bars. They are highly caustic. |
| Mottled soap with an irregular freckled look | ◆ Uneven stirring<br>◆ Fats or oils exposed to radical temperature changes during refinement or packaging | Proceed with process. This is an aesthetic problem only. |
| While cutting the few-days-old soap into bars, the knife meets with resistance in certain spots. Upon careful inspection, soaps have hard, shiny, white chunks of solid lye surrounding areas of normal soft soap and are wet underneath with a slippery liquid lye that soaks through the waxed-paper onto the soap frames. | ◆ Poured soap into frames before saponification was complete<br>◆ Stirring process too low and inconsistent | Do not use these bars — they are caustic. |
| Cracks in soaps | ◆ Too much sodium hydroxide<br>◆ Too much stirring, more like beating or whipping<br>◆ Soap set up too quickly | If these seem harsh, too much sodium hydroxide makes these unusable. If the cracks are temperature related, the problem is only an aesthetic one. |

## DIAGNOSING SIGNS OF TROUBLE IN THE FINAL SOAPS (CONT'D.)

| Trouble Sign | Reasons Why | What to Do |
|---|---|---|
| Soap takes over three days to harden considerably (following the covered insulation period) | ◆ Not enough sodium hydroxide<br>◆ Citrus oils slowing down the process slightly<br>◆ Curing soap exposed to extreme temperatures and/or drafts<br>◆ High percentage of castor oil with an insufficient amount of sodium hydroxide<br>◆ High percentage of unsaponified oils in soap formula | Allow the bars a few more weeks to cure. Do not use them if they never firm up sufficiently. |
| Lye pockets (air bubbles filled with liquid or powdered lye) | ◆ Insufficient stirring<br>◆ Too much sodium hydroxide<br>◆ Stirring process too slow | These bars are unsafe — the pockets of lye will burn. |

# CHAPTER 9
## Answers to Soapmakers' Most-Asked Questions

I have come by the following questions quite naturally — first, by asking them myself, and then by having them asked of me by others. It does not take long before beginners ask the hard questions. Some are philosophical. Some are scientific or technical. Some have clear answers, and some are controversial. In this chapter, I attempt to answer forty-one questions that have come my way more than once.

Natural vs. synthetic

Q: *Is the distinction between natural and synthetic a meaningful one?*

A: I think so, but some people want to know what all the fuss is about. Since everything in this world is a chemical, and since synthetic imitations are often structurally identical to natural compounds, why must we make a distinction? A pure essential oil contains quantifiable compounds, and if these components can be perfectly reproduced down to the last molecule, then why distinguish between the two end products?

You may sense in me a bias against synthetic perfection. I suppose I do have an underlying assumption that many more natural materials are understood and beneficial, while more synthetic things have unknown consequences. (Of course, some of the most toxic substances in this world are found in nature.) The fear of proven side effects, as well as of the unknown, leads me to avoid too many synthetic imitations. In this light, the preference for natural makes good sense. It is nothing more than the prudent person's reasonable avoidance of unnecessary risk.

Others see no reason to avoid technological innovation. They acknowledge the value of certain natural materials, but they consider purity, availability, and expense when choosing a synthetic reproduction over the natural option. "I've been eating red M&Ms my entire life and I haven't died yet" is persuasive to many. Common sense tells these folks that limited use — even of bad things — cannot cause much damage.

Some controversies involve a clear-cut right and wrong, but most don't. Not all natural materials are superior to synthetics, and not all synthetics are dangerous. We must make choices on a case-by-case basis. Some natural materials are safer and more effective than their synthetic counterparts, but some natural compounds are helpful when used medicinally in small doses and harmful in excess. Other natural materials are filled with impurities, and by the time they've been made safe for use, they've been refined in a variety of ways that leave them no better than the synthetic versions. On the other hand, some synthetic materials are dangerous whether or not they have been approved for use by some governmental agency.

We will all absorb some amount of unhealthy materials throughout our lifetimes, knowingly and unknowingly. The challenge is to remain alert to the options and to make informed choices.

Q: *What does it mean to "superfat" a soap?*

Superfatted formulas

A: The percentage of sodium hydroxide in a formula is carefully calculated according to the degree of saponification desired. When enough sodium hydroxide is used to supply all of the fatty acids with sodium hydroxide mates, the soap is considered fully saponified. No discount (see chapter 13, pages 244–245) is taken from the percentage of sodium hydroxide required for complete saponification. This fully saponified soap does not contain excess oils. By using less sodium hydroxide than is required for a complete saponification, however, fat and oil molecules run out of lye mates. The excess oil remains in the final bar of soap as a soothing moisturizer. This milder soap is called superfatted soap — it was provided with excess fat and oil to make it more moisturizing.

Nearly all bath soaps clean, but the degree of saponification determines how gently or how harshly they do their jobs. An excess of sodium hydroxide not only can strip the skin of dirt and excess oils, but it can take away important natural oils as well. People with dry skin are especially affected by the strip-clean. When emollient fats and oils are added to soap as superfatting ingredients, they lay a hydrophobic film on the skin's surface that softens the skin by holding in internal moisture.

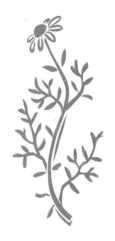

Q: *Can good mild soap be made without applying a sodium hydroxide discount?*

A: The most cleansing soap of all is produced without discounting (reducing) the amount of sodium hydroxide required for complete saponification. This soap better resists rancidity, since it has no excess oils to spoil. All of the molecules participating in the soapmaking reaction combine to make soap, with none left over to roam free. A fully saponified soap contains only soap — no excess lye and no excess fats and oils. It is the soap that cleans, not the lye and not the fats and oils. The excess oils in superfatted soap soothe, but they do not clean. A full saponification produces the most effective cleanser.

Though I still feel that a superfatted soap is milder, a fully saponified soap can also be mild. In theory, when a fully saponified formula is perfectly blended, there will be no excess lye present in the final bars. The soap is only slightly more alkaline than superfatted soap, since most soaps stubbornly cling to a pH of around 10 (see chapter 13, page 245) despite our clever enticements. The skin seems to adjust to this range.

The trouble with fully saponified formulas relates to processing, not to a faulty theory. Superfatted formulas build in a margin for error; fully saponified soap requires exactness. When the lye completely reacts with the oils, a fully saponified soap can be mild, but any lye that is not well incorporated precipitates out of solution in the form of solid or liquid lye in the final bars. Some soapmakers are better than others at ensuring that all of the lye reacts with all of the oils. As important as the quick-stir is for all formulas, the nondiscounted formula must be perfectly blended to avoid excess lye in the final bars. I find that even a quick, forceful hand-stir does not always incorporate all of the lye; only a machine-stir accomplishes this. I also recommend slightly higher soapmaking temperatures for better solubility. Soapmakers who make fully saponified soap note that though the soap occasionally feels slick just out of the molds, it becomes progressively milder during the three- to four-week cure period.

I continue to superfat my soap for the moisturizing effect of the extra dose of oils, and because the processing is more reliable, not because pH is dramatically affected. Highly alkaline sodium hydroxide and only slightly acidic vegetable oils react to form soap that is alkaline, not neutral. Though I have never overvalued pH, it seems prudent to add an excess of superfatting oils in an effort to keep it closer to the midrange of acceptable values (though still alkaline).

Should you prefer a more fully saponified soap to my more discounted formulas, begin with a 2 to 5 percent discount rather than taking no discount at all. This will leave some small percentage of emollient oils in the final bars.

Q: *How vigorously should a soap batch be stirred?*

*Stirring*

A: How quickly and thoroughly a soap mixture is stirred determines how quickly the components react to make soap. Though there are many different soapmaking methods, a cold-process soap should be stirred briskly and forcefully.

Soap is an excellent emulsifier for oil-in-water emulsions. It actually helps make itself. In the first phase of soapmaking, the oil globules are evenly dispersed in the lye. Some soap must form before there is enough to act as a catalyst — to help emulsify the rest of the oil/lye mixture. This soap helps to pull the rest of the mixture into the saponification process. Agitation from the start increases the rate of the reaction. Consistent, quick stirring keeps more yet-to-connect molecules in contact with one another, and it keeps the already saponified soap well dispersed in the unsaponified mixture. The soap mixture experiences a slowdown in its saponification rate after the initial activity, but continuous, quick strokes keep the soap smooth and intact until the next phase of the process begins.

When stirring by hand, stir as quickly as possible. In *The Natural Soap Book*, I qualified my instruction to stir quickly with "do not beat or whip." I have come to believe since then that it is impossible to stir too quickly by hand. Mechanical mixers, it is true, might go too fast. Heavy-duty mixers, hand-held mixers, blenders, and drills with paint-stirring attachments, when set at their medium to high speeds, can whip air bubbles into the soap mixture that will remain within the final bars and prevent a uniform texture. If you use a mixer, then, begin at setting 1; you can eventually increase to setting 2 when using a freestanding electric mixer. By hand, just go for it and work up a sweat. Stir hard, knowing that a quick saponification time is your reward.

To permit a quicker stir, choose a large soapmaking pan with plenty of headspace to accommodate the occasional splash of a forceful stir. A small pan filled close to the brim with soap will inhibit your speed, because you will fear splashing the mixture.

When you first add the lye to the oils, the mixture will be too thin and watery for an all-out beating. Still, stir as briskly as possible. About five minutes of continuous, quick stirring produces a thicker, more uniform mixture that can gradually tolerate faster and stronger strokes. From this point until the soap is ready to be poured, your stirring pattern should be continuous, forceful, and brisk, and should reach all corners of the soapmaking pan. Those who make soap in glass containers have seen for themselves the relationship between saponification time and the stirring rate. Through the glass, they literally see the separated oils and lye blending into one uniform, stable, thicker mixture.

Do not be concerned with stirring in a set pattern, such as a figure-eight design. There is nothing wrong with such a design and I often recommend it — but really just as a reminder to keep all of the soap in constant motion. Be sure to reach all corners of the pan in order to pull all players into the game. The full incorporation of materials produces a well-saponified soap. During the final few minutes before the soap is ready to be poured, you will find that the soap is thick enough to beat in random motions until the trace becomes evident.

*Allow adequate headspace in your soapmaking pan so you can stir as quickly as possible, keeping the entire mixture in motion.*

## Q: *Can I use blenders and mixers instead of hand-stirring?*

A: This is a matter of preference. Many people make soap using some mechanical advantage, but I like to be more intimately involved in the stirring process, and I enjoy the workout. My five-pound experimental batches are all made in the KitchenAid, but I hand-stir all of my 12 pound and larger batches. The needs of people dictate innovation, and just as some worship the microwave, others are thankful for attachments and mixers that take over the lion's share of the stirring.

All stir styles can make good soap provided the speed is fast enough. Since a brisk, forceful stir shortens the tracing time, mixers and brisk hand-stirring produce soap more quickly than does a leisurely stir. Quick, consistent strokes produce smooth soap with a fine grain and less risk of incomplete saponification. The small batches in this book are perfectly suited to the freestanding mixer. All soap that incorporates a high percentage of milk is best produced in a mixer; the cream is more finely dispersed by the consistent, fast speed and you will end up with a less grainy soap.

Those who prefer mixers to the spatula use heavy-duty kitchen mixers, large industrial mixers, a drill with a paint-stirring attachment, or even the kitchen blender. The only one of these I warn against is the blender. Those who use it swear by it, but be careful. I have accidentally sprayed fruits and vegetables across the room and have no reason to believe that the same couldn't happen with harsh, raw soap. Splashes can occur with hand-stirring and with any mechanical stir, but blenders have minds of their own and make all of the decisions. Some inexpensive blenders do not have tightly fitting lids; they weren't designed to make soap. Also, blenders produce soap with loads of air bubbles that may remain in the final bars.

Handheld mixers also carry their share of risk. They are difficult to control. For those who want to use a mixer, I recommend the freestanding type with an extra bowl, paddle, and splash-guard dedicated only to soapmaking to avoid contamination.

## Q: How does warm weather affect saponification?

A: Many soapmakers complain about slower tracing times during the summer months, especially those who live in humid areas. This makes some sense. The amount of water in a formula is directly related to the processing time and to the time the bars take to evaporate excess moisture.

On hot, humid days, the air contains more moisture. Normally, when air is less dense, it can absorb moisture from its surroundings — for example, from a curing soap that is trying to release its excess moisture from within. During soapmaking, the saponifying mixture contains a high percentage of glycerin, a humectant that attracts water from the air. Just as bars of glycerin soap draw moisture to their surface in the form of condensation on humid days, a soap mixture with glycerin attracts water from a humid environment, and the environment allows practically no evaporation. This extra water overloads the mixture and lengthens its tracing time.

If you make soap in hot, moist conditions, decrease your water percentages slightly and be most conscientious about a quick, firm stirring process.

## Q: Why does soap need to be covered during the cure?

A: Saponification is a chemical reaction that can take place in a closed vessel, in an open pot, in a vacuum, or on your fingertips. The coming together and the reaction of certain chemicals produces soap; the reaction is not a terribly particular one. Ideally, cold-process soap is made using carefully calculated percentages of fats and oils, water, and sodium hydroxide; a general range of temperatures; a brisk stir; a short, covered cure at warm temperatures; and, finally, a cooler, dark, dry cure of a few weeks. But soap can be made in far less than ideal circumstances.

You can cheat on the eighteen- to twenty-four-hour insulation period, but for optimum results, don't. The warm insulation period allows further saponification to take place, prevents separation, and may control the amount of residue that forms on the surface of the soap.

Even soap made at 80°F (27°C) warms up further during the insulation period — usually to around 90°F (32°C). The range of soapmaking temperatures (80–120°F, or 27–49°C) produces soap that stays warm enough under cover to continue the saponification process. Soap is only partially saponified when it is poured into molds; most of the remainder of the reaction takes place over the next few days, and the final bit of curing takes place over the next few weeks. Soap is continually becoming more and more saponified and, therefore, more and more mild. This is what the aging process is all about. My soap and I mellow with age.

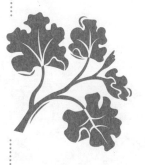

Another reason to cover freshly poured soap is to avoid separation. Excess fats and oils, nutrients, and essential oils separate out of solution at extreme high and low temperatures. Soap made using cooler temperatures (80–85°F, or 27–29.4°C) can tolerate a quicker cool-down than can soap made at higher temperatures (100–150°F, or 38–65.5°C). Separation is more likely to occur in those batches made at high temperatures and cooled too quickly. Soap processed at any temperature has a better opportunity to complete the saponification process and avoid separation when it is covered for close to a day.

With each skipped step comes some risk of throwing the reaction off track. The overall process can tolerate some creative license (I've made good soap that was only insulated for six to eight hours), but not too much. Temperatures, cure time, and stirring can be adjusted, but each adjustment alters the final soap in some small way, and though the final product can be clearly identified as soap, the texture, smell, and integrity of the product will be affected in some small or large way. So, yes, the warmer cure period can be ignored, and your final soap may even be close to what you could have achieved, but — depending upon the particular formula and the particular process — it may not be as desirable.

**Q:** *How critical are the insulation period and the following three weeks of curing?*

**A:** Cold-process saponification is a long process that stretches over a two- to three-week period. When soap is poured into molds, it has only partially saponified; even hard, week-old bars of soap are still busy tying up loose ends. When the soap has traced, perhaps 40 to 50 percent of the mixture has saponified. A warm insulation period of eighteen to twenty-four hours encourages the further reaction of molecules; too quick a cooling slows this activity and could leave an imbalanced blend, even after a few weeks of air-curing. I have unwrapped perfectly good soap after only eight hours, but most formulas benefit from the additional time under wraps.

The two- to three-week air-cure is important for two reasons. First, as saponification continues, the soap becomes progressively milder. And second, as the water in the soap evaporates, the soap becomes harder and longer-lasting.

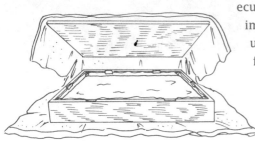

During the insulation period, the soap in the tray continues to saponify.

**Q:** *How does climate affect curing?*

**A:** Just after you pour freshly made soap, the mixture ideally needs a warm, closed, dry environment to complete the saponification process. Soap can be made in a less-than-ideal setting, but aim to comply with as many of the ideal conditions as possible. Once uncovered, after eighteen hours, a cold-process superfatted soap cures best in a dry, temperate (60–70°F, or 15.5–21°C) environment.

Cold-process soap retains the glycerin produced during the chemical reaction, as well as some of the excess water used to make the soap. You allow the soap to cure for a few weeks to give it time to release this excess moisture content through evaporation. But a conflicting process occurs as the water evaporates. Cold-process soaps contain free glycerin, a humectant that attracts moisture, and as water evaporates from the soap, the free glycerin attracts new moisture from the environment.

Therefore, the curing environment should be dry, to encourage evaporation and discourage the attraction of additional moisture. Remember that the curing cold-process soap acts as a sponge, so it is important to limit the potential sources of moisture. A dry setting allows for the release of internal moisture along with preventing the absorption of external moisture.

Q: *How much water should I use?*

Water

A: The water in a soapmaking formula carries the sodium hydroxide to all corners of the pan, then participates in a process called hydrolysis — the splitting of the neutral fats and oils into fatty acids and glycerin. Fats and oils cannot react with sodium hydroxide to make soap; only their components can. So water and sodium hydroxide together, in the lye solution, split apart the fats and oils. Throughout the soapmaking process, the water evaporates. Most soap mixtures only retain about 15 percent of the water added at the start.

Old soap formulas often do not separately itemize sodium hydroxide and water. Instead, they list a lye solution in degrees Baumé. For years, soapmakers used an aqueous solution of sodium carbonate or potassium carbonate, until it was discovered how to easily produce sodium hydroxide (the carbonates were reacted with other chemicals to produce a hydroxide solution that was stronger than its original carbonates). This stronger lye solution served soapmakers well until sodium hydroxide became accessible. The Baumé scale (written as Bé in notation) was named for Antoine Baumé and measures specific gravity in degrees; within soapmaking, it measures the concentration of the lye solution by comparing the density of the sodium hydroxide to the density of the water. Since temperature is related to density, measurements vary depending upon the temperature of the water. Without getting too detailed, each degree Baumé at a particular temperature corresponds with a specific percentage by weight of sodium hydroxide. A 38°Bé lye solution at 60°F (15.5°C) is approximately 32 percent by weight NaOH, which translates to 2 ounces (56.7 g) of sodium hydroxide in 4.25 ounces (120.48 g) of water. Note that the number of degrees Bé does not equal the percentage of NaOH; 38°Bé means 32 percent NaOH, not 38 percent NaOH. Of course, the Bé scale is only a general rule, since the strength of the solution varies as fats and oils change, as well as soapmaking temperatures. Instruments called hydrometers measure the specific gravity of the lye solution.

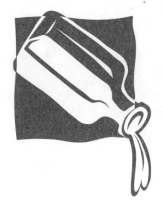

Modern soap formulas, including mine, typically do not refer to Bé solutions. Instead, NaOH and water are listed separately. Soap formulas must balance the percentages of fats and oils, water, and sodium hydroxide. Additional ingredients must not offset this balance. The percentage of water is directly related to the amount of sodium hydroxide; it is also directly related to the total weight of the fats and oils and to the soapmaking temperatures. Soap made at higher temperatures requires slightly more water because of the loss to evaporation; again, most soap mixtures only retain about 15 percent of the water added at the start. A good general rule is 6 ounces (170 g) of water for every 1 pound (400 g) of fats and oils.

Most turn-of-the-century soap formulas use a 30 percent lye solution. Though the soapmaking process was very different then, 30 percent is still a good starting point. Remember that the arithmetic follows a certain order. First you calculate the amount of sodium hydroxide that you need, which depends entirely upon the amount of fats and oils and their SAP values (see chapter 13, page 247). Then you calculate the amount of water by dividing the weight of NaOH by three-tenths (.3). This will yield the total weight of the NaOH-plus-water. Subtracting the weight of the NaOH gives you the weight of water you must add. For example, 2 ounces of NaOH would require a lye solution weighing 6.67 ounces (2 ÷ .3), which means that 4.67 ounces of water must be added (6.67 ounces total − 2 ounces NaOH).

For superfatting soaps, the strength of the lye solution doesn't change — only your quantity of oils does.

## Q: Why use distilled water?

A: Someday, future generations may laugh at us for purchasing bottled water that is often comparable to what comes out of the tap. Certain areas of the world do have horrible water, filled with impurities. But some people have access to delicious local water — yet buy what was already given to them, relegating the gift to flushing, bathing, swimming, and watering.

Most of the time, tap water is fine for making soap. I recommend the use of distilled water, however, because many people do not know if their water is pure and soft. As I've said so often, a few pieces of the soap-making puzzle can be missing without ruining the final product, but I try to begin close to the ideal, knowing that nature and I will fall a little short by the end.

Pure, soft water contributes to pure soap. Contaminated water affects the integrity of the soap, though few of us have this degree of contamination. Hard water contains dissolved mineral salts that react with the sodium hydroxide ions in the lye solution, leaving fewer of these ions to make soap during the saponification process. The lye is sapped of some of its strength.

Though it is tough to know how pure bottled water is, experience is the best test. I could be misplacing my trust when I assume that the bottled water contains fewer impurities — perhaps it is no softer than tap. Still, these are the assumptions I make. One day I may pay for laboratory testing and do my own comparisons.

## Q: Can batch size be reduced or increased without affecting ingredient proportions?

Changing batch size

A: Though keeping ingredient proportions consistent seems intuitively reasonable, things are not quite that simple. The less cooperative factors are water and temperature. Some formulas can be halved or doubled by dividing or multiplying the ingredients accordingly, but the percentage of water may require a slight adjustment. Smaller batches may also require slightly higher processing temperatures to ensure a complete saponification (see chapter 7).

Cold-process saponification is dependent upon the correct balance of neutral oils and sodium hydroxide. If this balance remains intact, a batch can be divided or multiplied without affecting saponification. But saponification — the chemical reaction that produces soap — is not the only determining factor. The amount of moisture in the final bars determines a soap's hardness and texture. Too much water produces a soft soap; too little water produces a dry soap prone to cracking.

How much or how little water is left in the final bars is directly related to the curing environment, and to the surface area and temperature used to make the soap. If you quarter a formula but make the soap with about the same-sized pan and at the same (or a warmer) temperature as the larger batch, more water evaporates during the saponification process. The final bars are not as plastic and moist as those the original formula would have produced. Those soapmakers who make soap at warmer temperatures must pay special attention to heat and evaporation; otherwise, their final bars are too dry.

Q: *What is the white powder on the surface of pretrimmed soap?*

A: This is the million-dollar question. I don't know for certain what this substance is. After the insulation period, many batches have a light dusting of white powder on the exposed surface of the soap (to be differentiated from a heavy coating of powdery residue, which is due to an excess of sodium hydroxide). I had always read and been told (and passed along in *The Natural Soap Book*) that this substance was sodium carbonate, the result of free sodium hydroxide reacting with carbon dioxide in the air. I accepted this explanation and never thought about it again until I noticed some unusual patterns.

For one thing, some batches of soap produce little or no "soda ash," another name for the sodium carbonate; soaps with high percentages of cocoa butter, beeswax, or castor oil are often residue-free. For another, the same formula can produce less residue one day than it does the next.

Powdery residue on soap

And the same formula processed at different soapmaking temperatures, or in smaller or larger batches, produces soap with varying amounts of residue. Certain essential and fragrance oils also affect the production of residue. If the residue is sodium carbonate — related only to free alkali — then the above findings make no sense.

The more I poke and prod, the less I feel that this residue is sodium carbonate. Of course, this is the opinion of a layperson. I have asked a few chemists whether this substance could simply be dried soap. The glycerin in a cold-process soap makes the soap hydroscopic, meaning that it attracts water; it is possible that the soap molecules closest to the air draw moisture from the air and dry as fine crystals of soap, redeposited on the surface of the soap mass. It makes some sense to me that different fats, oils, and nutrients react to moisture differently, dry differently, and produce different amounts of residue. It makes no sense to me that batches of soap that contain identical percentages of sodium hydroxide would react differently to the air and produce different quantities of sodium carbonate.

The powdery residue is sometimes harsher (burns more using the tongue-test, which involves a light touching of the tip of the tongue to the soap to test for harshness) than the rest of the soap; this is part of the reason that I so quickly accepted it as the base sodium carbonate. But powdered soap residue might also have a mild bite to it. Perhaps soap that precipitates into a powder is simply more basic, because it does not cure as fully as the whole bar does. Also, the bite is not meaningfully stronger than that of the underlying soap after a few days of curing. A few weeks later, neither the bar nor the residue is harsh. I would expect sodium carbonate to be harsh at any time.

Finally, after over five years of soapmaking, I asked a chemist to test the powder on a few of my bars for sodium carbonate. He found no trace of it. He agreed that the residue may be dried soap, and added that producing sodium carbonate is no easy task. In the lab, its production is a deliberate process, not a reaction that happens casually, by accident. Free alkali has a difficult time combining with the carbon dioxide in the air. In the case of rancidity, oxygen is champing at the bit to react with stray molecules. But it seems that carbon dioxide and

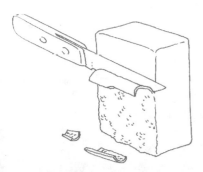

If the light powdery residue on your bars bothers you, it can be sliced off.

sodium are not so inclined to react with one another — to the contrary, a monumental effort might be required to force the union.

I still do not know for sure what this powdery residue on the surface of some bars is. But I'm intrigued by the question, and as more chemists support my hunch with scientific know-how, I'm led to believe that the light dusting is not so harsh after all. Slice it off if it bothers you, but after a few weeks of curing, this residue seems to be as mild as the rest of the soap.

Q: *How can I avoid the residue — whatever it actually is?*

A: Whether the light dusting of powder is sodium carbonate, dry soap, or something else, the more pressing question is, "Can it be avoided?" I have found that it can. My soap produces very little residue — sometimes none.

Certain fats and oils produce more of this residue than others during saponification. I find very little residue when I make formulas that include castor oil, beeswax, or cocoa butter. Also, soap that stays warm during the insulation process does not dry as quickly, and this results in less residue. Allow the soap eighteen to twenty-four hours under cover. The percentage of water seems related to the formation of this powder as well; too little water causes a quicker drying reaction and more powder.

The powdery residue is heaviest when it forms during the first twenty-four hours after the soap is poured. The drying reaction may be stage-driven, such that controlling when the surface of the soap dries out will allow you to control how much or how little residue forms. The goal is to keep the soap's surface moist for the first day; after that, less and less residue forms as the surface finally dries.

Should your favorite formula be a stickler, you can use the following techniques to trick it into cooperation, if you consider the residue worth the fuss. (I don't.) I always line my trays with heavy-duty waxed paper, and I have found that laying a piece of this paper directly on the surface of the bars (waxed-side down) immediately after I poured the soap reduces the powder — often entirely. (Microwave plastic wrap and plastic trash bags work as well, but the plastic is prone to sticking, so I prefer heavy-duty waxed paper.)  The paper can be removed after a day or so, because the reaction that forms the powder seems to be phase-driven — the chemical reaction takes place only during a particular phase of the soapmaking process. The powder forms during the first eighteen hours under cover or not at all.

I once experimented and covered only a small portion of the soap's surface with this paper immediately after I poured the soap into the tray. Following the insulation period, the exposed soap had a light dusting of powder, while the soap beneath the waxed paper was free of it. Thinking that the paper may only have delayed the eventual formation of this powder, I peeled off the paper and left the soap to cure. The powder never formed. I'm led to believe that whatever its cause, the chemical reaction that creates the powder is limited to a particular phase of the soapmaking process during which it must take place — or it will never take place.

The heavy-duty waxed paper acts as a barrier between the soap and the environment. In theory, no extra reactions can take place. Since my soaps form so little of this powder, I don't bother with the extra layer of paper. But those who routinely experience a more significant buildup may want to try to prevent it.

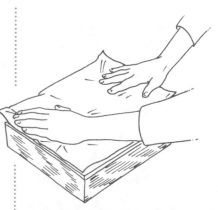

If you are really **determined** to prevent the powdery residue from forming on your bars, try placing a piece of heavy-duty waxed paper directly on the surface of the bars (waxed-side down) immediately after pouring the soap.

Q: *What are the flecks that sometimes float on the surface of the lye solution?*

Flecks in lye

A: Sodium hydroxide reacts with carbon dioxide in the air to form what may be sodium carbonate, which does not dissolve into the larger lye solution. Cooler conditions are most favorable for this chemical reaction. This sodium carbonate is visible as what I call "lye lint," specks of crystals that float on the surface of the cooling lye. This residue does not affect the quality of the final soap. The pieces of "lint" are incorporated during the soapmaking process and are indistinguishable within the final bars. All soap contains some sodium carbonate — the diluted, milder form of sodium hydroxide.

Another thing to keep in mind is that sodium hydroxide varies in purity from lot to lot and company to company. All sodium hydroxide contains some carbonate. The higher grades keep this percentage to a figure that does not affect soapmaking but still produce varying degrees of lye lint.

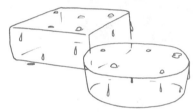

Sweating soap

Moisture on the surface of soap is actually condensation from the air.

## Q: Why does soap sweat?

A: During a normal curing period, soap releases a percentage of its water to the air when there is less water in the air than there is in the soap. The water within the bar migrates to the surface before evaporating into the air. This is how soap dries and becomes harder. When the amount of water in the air is higher than the amount in the soap, a glycerin soap attracts the external moisture to its surface in the form of condensation. Before evaporation, water in soap works its way from deep inside the bar, where the water content is highest, to the drier surface, where there is less water. Thus curing soap undergoes two opposing reactions: The glycerin in the soap attracts water from the environment to the soap, and the water inside the soap gradually evaporates. Atmospheric conditions affect these processes.

Hot, humid conditions almost always cause small beads of condensation. They are a nuisance, but also a telltale sign of the purity of a soap.

Glycerin is a humectant, meaning that it is moisturizing because it attracts and holds moisture, releasing it gradually. Cold-process soap retains the glycerin created during the soapmaking process and creates a more moisturizing bar. But the same glycerin that balances the skin's moisture content is also a magnet for any moisture in the air. This moisture is drawn to the surface of the bar, condenses, and stays put until it is wiped off or until the air is dry enough to allow evaporation. With enough humidity, the glycerin is so effective that it can reach moisture through the confines of fabric or paper, leaving limp packaging.

Depending upon the degree of saponification and superfatting of a particular soap, its integrity may or may not be affected by moisture. A fully saponified soap can tolerate wetness better than a soap chock-full of creamy oils and nutrients. To avoid the fuss, store your soap in dry, cool, dark areas. Wet soaps can be dealt with, and soap can be stored in less-than-ideal surroundings, but try for the ideal.

**Q:** *Should I scrape clean the sides of the soapmaking pan while I pour the soap?*

Scraping sides of pan

**A:** Beginners should avoid scraping the sides of the soapmaking pan while pouring the soap into molds. It is better to leave behind a few tablespoons of unblended mixture than to pollute your batch. But after making many batches of soap, you will have learned to keep all of the soap mixture in motion, including the buildup on the sides of the pan. If, during the stir process, the sides of the pan are periodically scraped and incorporated into the blend, the soap clinging to the sides will be the same mixture as the rest of the batch.

However, you should always avoid scraping the sides of the pan if a powdery residue has collected at soap level. This means that your stirring has been irregular. It is good to minimize waste, but the buildup should not be included if it appears grainy.

**Q:** *Can soap be better unmolded by freezing it first?*

Unmolding

**A:** When stubborn batches of soap will not release from plastic molds, some soapmakers pop the molds into the freezer for a half hour or so. When the cold soap is then placed in a room-temperature space, it sweats. The slippery soap then releases easily from the mold.

I feel like a party pooper, but I don't recommend this technique for removal. I have yet to test a previously frozen bar that compared favorably to one traditionally cured. The frozen soap soon thaws and continues to cure, but the texture is often somewhat slimy, grainy, or crumbly. Just as ice crystals degrade ice cream, they seem to affect soap. I also have a feeling that the interrupted saponification process never quite gets back on track. Of course, ice cream that has undergone a thaw and refreeze is still edible (though not as good), and soap that has been frozen will still clean and moisturize. But since my soapmaking is time-consuming and costly, I'd rather not cut unnecessary corners in the last step. While freezing soap is an option, and many soapmakers swear by it, I choose to skip any mold that causes such a fuss.

Sodium hydroxide ............▶

## Q: *Which form of sodium hydroxide should I use?*

A: Sodium hydroxide can be purchased as beads, flakes, or liquid (already dissolved in water). The liquid is impractical unless the manufacturer is around the corner, you own a pickup truck, and you've got friends with good strong backs. The cost of shipping sodium hydroxide in solution is prohibitive. Also, when you purchase liquid sodium hydroxide, you must adapt the measurements in your formula to accommodate the strength of that particular lye solution.

Beads are the familiar form sold as lye in the supermarket — tiny pearls that are easily dissolved in water. Some soapmakers also like the flakes that can be purchased from chemical supply houses. The flat flakes (they look like quick oats) stay put a little better than the beads, which cling to plastic and spill more haphazardly.

Choose whichever form — flakes or beads — is more easily accessible, since chemically they are nearly identical. Both usually contain around the same percentage of sodium hydroxide, and their percentages of other active ingredients and trace elements are also comparable. Some companies offer a higher-grade sodium hydroxide than you really need, with fewer impurities. This grade is overkill for soapmaking, and the cost is much higher than what you would ordinarily pay.

flakes

beads

## Q: *Can another base be substituted for sodium hydroxide?*

A: People often ask if soap can be made without using sodium hydroxide. The answer is yes, but the alternatives are no more desirable as raw materials — often less desirable. This is one synthetic chemical that is the better choice.

An acid and a base must combine to produce soap. The acid is usually a neutral oil or a pure fatty acid. The base can vary, but only sodium hydroxide is well suited to the cold-process soapmaking method. Sea salts from an alkaline lake such as the Dead Sea may contain some potassium salts that are alkaline enough to produce soap — but if they are, they are also nearly as harsh as sodium hydroxide, so nothing is gained. No weak alkali can replace sodium hydroxide when making a cold-process soap.

There are, however, many substances that have soaplike properties, though they cannot replace sodium hydroxide in our soapmaking recipes. The roots, bark, leaves, seeds, or fruits of a variety of plants contain saponin, an alkali-free substance that lathers and cleans in a primitive way. Many of the following release a thin lather when mashed:

- **Sea-snail eggs.** Sailors and fishermen gather these small yellow eggs, which they call sea-washballs, to clean themselves. They are found on the ocean floor.
- **Soap apple.** The bulbs of this lilylike plant yield a thick lather with a soapy smell that cleans fairly well.
- **Soapbark.** The soapbark tree belongs to the rose family; its bark is used as soap.
- **Soapberry.** This tree grows in Spain and tropical America. Its roots are mashed into a pulp for a soaplike lather.
- **Soapwort (bouncing bet).** This plant's leaves produce a soaplike lather when mashed with water.
- **Spanish bayonet.** This was used to clean by Native Americans.
- **Yucca.** This plant was used as a cleanser by Native Americans.

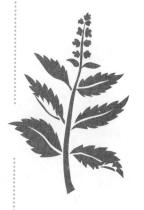

## Q: *Why is too much coconut oil in a formula drying to the skin?*

Coconut oil

A: Coconut oil is a wonderful soapmaking oil, but it should be limited to around 30 percent of the total soapmaking fats and oils. Fatty-acid chains that contain twelve or fewer carbon atoms are more acidic than fatty-acid chains with more carbon atoms. These more acidic fatty acids clean well, but can be drying when overused.

The reason is that $C_{12}$ chains remove more of the skin's natural oil. The acid mantle on our skin's surface is a layer of oil that protects by serving as a barrier. Coconut, palm kernel, and babassu oil soaps remove this oil, because the fatty ends of these soap molecules match the skin's oil and quickly latch onto it. The soap molecule emulsifies and suspends this oil, leaving the skin without this layer of protection.

Any excess coconut oil left on the now basic site (without its acidic raincoat) releases protons there and irritates the skin. The skin pretty much says, "I don't like that proton there," and gets dry and red.

When coconut oil makes up 20 to 30 percent of a soap formula, it offers a wonderful lather, and in the company of other less acidic fats and oils, such as olive and palm oil, it is not drying. But when coconut oil is used as a majority percentage of a formula, it can irritate more sensitive individuals.

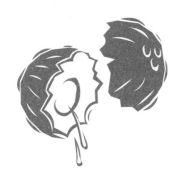

Q: *Is there a practical difference between coconut oil and palm kernel oil?*

A: Coconut oil and palm kernel oil are chemically alike and can be used interchangeably in a soap formula. They both contain high percentages of the shorter-chain fatty acids, lauric acid and myristic acid ($C_{12}$ and $C_{14}$), and similar percentages of all of their fatty acids. Coconut oil has slightly more lauric acid, and palm kernel oil has slightly more myristic acid.

The chemistry is such that variations in the percentages of different fatty acids account for differences among fats and oils and their soaps. Both lauric acid and myristic acid produce hard bars with quick, fluffy lathers, but myristic acid is slightly less irritating and lauric acid produces a slightly fuller lather. Of course, these two fatty acids are so closely related that any distinction is subtle. Because coconut oil and palm kernel oil contain only slightly more or less of these two fatty acids, their soaps are not meaningfully different.

Within a carefully designed soap formula, I have been unable to distinguish between these two oils (or babassu oil, which shares a similar makeup but is hardest of the three to locate). Use whichever is most accessible and reasonably priced — which will most often be coconut.

Q: *Can all kinds of milk be used to make soap?*

A: Milk soap can be made using buttermilk, goat's milk, powdered milk, coconut milk, or 2 percent, skim, or homogenized cow's milk — basically, any milk. Soapmakers often prefer one milk over another. I find that the heavier blends contribute a richer feel to the final bars than does skim milk, which has a lower fat content and a higher percentage of water. My favorites are goat's milk and buttermilk, because they have richer textures and contain more fat and less water; I think that I notice this in the final soap. The various kinds of milk may not be meaningfully different from one another, however, so use the kind that is most convenient.

Milk is secreted by the mammary glands of female mammals as nourishment for their offspring. Depending upon the mammal, this liquid varies from opaque white to yellow. Milk consists of globules of butterfat, water, lactose (a milk sugar), casein (a group of proteins, pronounced *kay-'seen* or *'kay-see-en*), and salts. Milks differ most in their percentages of fat. Reindeer's milk contains the most fat, nearly six times that of cow's or goat's milk.

Whole milk is the milk from a cow before any reduction in fat has been made. The globules of fat are lighter than water and float to the top, forming cream. Whole milk contains about 3.25 percent of this cream. It can be forced through a sieve, which will break up and uniformly disperse the minuscule fat globules that would otherwise float on top. The resulting well-blended milk is called homogenized milk, and its cream content is also about 3.25 percent. When the percentage of cream is reduced to .5 percent or less, skim, nonfat, and low-fat milk are created; they contain the protein and mineral value of whole milk, but they lack the fat-soluble vitamins of whole milk, such as vitamins A, D, E, and K.

When the cream from milk is churned, the fat globules come together and compact into butter. Buttermilk is a by-product created during the churning process. Buttermilk is also made commercially by adding a culture to skim milk, and it often contains cream or butter. Powdered milk is made by pasteurizing milk and air-drying it to a 5 percent moisture content. Whole dry milk contains more fat than nonfat dry milk.

Be sure to whisk as quickly as possible when you add milk to the lye solution, to keep the components fairly well blended. The casein in milk dissolves in lye, but the cream (fat) reacts with some lye to form soap. Don't worry about any small lumps; they will be broken up and absorbed into the soap mixture later in the soapmaking process. I prefer to make milk soap using a freestanding electric mixer, because its lower settings do a better job than I do blending the lumps finely into the soap to create a creamy, uniform blend. When milk replaces all of the water in a formula, the resulting soap has a tendency to be grainier than one made using half water/half milk. I should mention that the smell of the lye/milk solution is bad, though it disappears in the final bars a day or so into the curing process.

Keep color in mind when you choose a variety of milk. Cow's milk is yellowish due to its carotene content, while the milk of ewes and goats is almost chalk white. These slight variations can lend shades of white, cream, and beige to the final bars, and they are all pretty. Milk soaps are often some shade of brown, as the milk/lye solution darkens most formulas. For lighter shades, minimize the amount of time that the milk is in contact with the lye solution before you combine it with the fats and oils; if you like darker brown shades, allow more time.

There are a couple of ways to incorporate the milk. When you are using it to replace all of the water, you can whisk the sodium hydroxide into it, just as you would normally add the sodium hydroxide to water. To avoid grainy, mottled milk soap, add the lye/milk mixture to room temperature fats and oils immediately after the lye dissolves. Aim for around 8 ounces (226.8 g) of milk per 1 pound (400 g) of fats and oils to compensate for the portion of the milk — the fat — that is lost to saponification. If you are using milk to replace half or less of the water, aim for 6 ounces (170 g) of water/milk mixture per 1 pound (400 g) of fats and oils.

I prefer part-milk/part-water to all-milk soap. When using part milk/part water, you can add the sodium hydroxide to the blended milk and water, or you can add it to the water only, adding the milk to the lye solution later — when the lye is ready to be mixed with the fats and oils. When I want white or cream-colored bars, I use part milk/part water and delay the addition of the milk to the lye (I warm the milk in the microwave first to the temperature of the lye solution) until the last moment. When I want warm caramel shades, I either use all milk, or I add the milk to the lye solution soon after the lye is dissolved. Whichever method I use, I whisk like mad in an effort to keep lumps to a minimum.

The soapmaking temperatures for milk soaps vary, depending upon which of the above procedures you use to incorporate the milk. When using all milk and no water, or when the milk and the lye cool for an hour or more, I find that slightly warmer temperatures (100–120°F [38–49°C] for the lye/milk and 90–100°F [32–38°C] for the fats and oils) do a better job of smoothing out the lumpy mixture. When I add the milk to the lye immediately before adding this lye/milk mixture to the fats and oils, I stay with my lower soapmaking temperatures (80–100°F, or 27–38°C).

Q: *What is grapefruit seed extract?*

*Natural preservatives*

A: In 1964, Dr. Jakob Harich, the president of Chemie Research and Manufacturing Company, Inc. (see "Suppliers" in the appendix), developed an extract from the ground seeds and membranes of the grapefruit that had antiseptic, antibiotic, and antioxidant properties. Medicinally, grapefruit seed extract is used to treat a variety of bacterial and viral infections, internally and externally, from skin wounds and dandruff to ear infections and infected throats.

Grapefruit seed extract can be used as an antioxidant to extend the shelf life of superfatted soap. As little as .5 percent (of the total soap-making ingredients) grapefruit seed extract is enough. A skin-care product that contains organic nutrients has a limited shelf life, since the organic materials work because they are metabolically active, and since anything alive is continually breaking down. Those soapmakers who choose mild, medicinal bars over more basic soap superfat their soaps and include organic nutrients in their formulas. They also accept a shorter shelf life as a sign of the soap's purity.

You have three options: to superfat your soap with excess oils and use, or not use, natural preservatives such as grapefruit seed extract; to take no discount from the amount of sodium hydroxide required for complete saponification, leaving your soap without the excess oils that will spoil over time; or to superfat your soap and use synthetic preservatives, many of which are suspect carcinogens. I choose the first option. All of my formulas list grapefruit seed extract as the antioxidant of choice, but you may or may not need it. If your favorite formulas contain a higher percentage of sodium hydroxide than mine, or fewer nutrients, or if a year or so of shelf life is plenty for your soapmaking needs, you will not need to purchase this expensive preservative. But if you share more of my particulars, grapefruit seed extract will extend the life of most of your soaps by a year or two, as well as contributing skin-care qualities of its own. Many soapmakers have told me that the addition of grapefruit seed extract decreases their tracing times meaningfully.

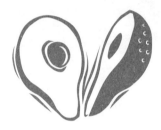

Q: *Is a preservative necessary?*

A: If a soap is superfatted, it contains a higher percentage of oils and fats than is needed to convert all of the sodium hydroxide into soap. This extra portion of neutral oils does not saponify. Instead, it is left as neutral oil or fatty acid within the final bars, and contributes mildness and emollience to the soap.

Superfatted soap is more prone to rancidity, however, since the unsaponified oils are less stable than the saponified product called soap. Soaps that contain active nutrients, such as honey or aloe vera gel, are also more likely to spoil, since organic matter breaks down as it completes its life cycle within the bar of soap.

Fully saponified soap is usually more harsh but may last for years without spoiling. Superfatted, organic soap degrades over time, but that does not mean that preservatives are imperative. The need for preservatives should be determined on a case-by-case basis.

Many factors come into play. Will the soap be used within a year or so? Does the bar contain a high percentage of unsaturated oils? Is the percentage of unsaponified fats and oils high? Is the soap for personal use or for sale to stores and customers? Does the soap already contain pure essential oils, herbal infusions, dried herbs, or other nutrients that contribute preservative properties of their own? Will the soap be exposed to warm, humid environments or repeated shifts in temperature?

If the soap will be used within six months, the high cost of natural preservatives is probably not merited. But if a superfatted bar is likely to experience life-shortening conditions as described above, a preservative such as grapefruit seed extract can extend shelf life while contributing its own share of skin-care qualities to the final bars.

## Q: *What is lecithin and can it be added to soap?*

Lecithin

A: Lecithin is a mixture of fatty acids found in all living cells, protecting the cells from oxidation and keeping them soft. Chemically, it is a phospholipid — an ester of glycerol that can be saponified. Whereas a triglyceride contains three fatty acids and glycerol, a phospholipid contains two fatty acids, glycerol, and a functional group derived from phosphoric acid. Lecithin, like soap, has a distinct head and tail that serve as surfactants. It is thought to help digest fats by dispersing them in water and carrying them out of the body, just as soap grabs hold of oily substances and holds them until the entire unit is washed away.

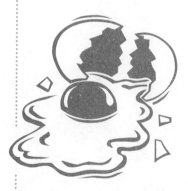

Lecithin is often obtained from soybeans or egg yolks, and occasionally from grains, fish, wheat germ, legumes, or brewer's yeast. As a fatty substance, it is used in cosmetics as an emollient, an antioxidant, and a thickener. Lecithin can be included in a soap formula. Since it saponifies, it can be added to the fats and oils at the start of the soapmaking process, but I add it at the trace since it can thicken the mixture before the oils and the lye have reacted sufficiently. Limit the quantity of lecithin used in a soap formula to 1 tablespoon (15 ml) per 1 pound (453.6 g) of soap, since — as an emulsifier — it can cause a premature emulsion, before a true trace has been achieved.

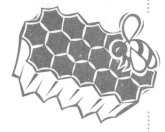

## Q: *What does honey contribute to soap?*

A: Many varieties of bees produce this sweet syrup from the nectar in flowers; they secrete the honey to build their cells and provide for winter sustenance. Honey is a mixture of plant nectar and bee enzymes. The color and taste of honey depend upon the flower from which the nectar was obtained; particular plants lend distinctive flavors and colors to their honey. All honey contains large quantities of enzymes; a hormone; carbohydrates; B-complex vitamins; vitamins C, D, and E; and some minerals. Temperatures above 100°F (38°C) destroy these active ingredients, so only add honey at the trace, and use lower-range soapmaking temperatures.

Honey lays down a clear, protective film that helps skin maintain moisture. It hydrates and soothes the skin and is thought to be slightly antiseptic and bacteriostatic. It does all of this without being greasy, even contributing astringent value. It is used as an emollient in soap. To avoid overloading a batch of soap (excess will ooze out of solution), add no more than 2 teaspoons (10 ml) of honey per 1 pound (400 g) of soap.

## Q: *When, why, and how should bee propolis be added to soap?*

A: Bees do not make propolis; rather, they collect this resinous material from plants, and use it along with beeswax to construct their hives. To beekeepers, it is known as "bee glue." Various studies suggest that propolis is antibacterial, reduces inflammation, and stimulates the immune system.

Solid propolis is available in 90 percent and 100 percent concentrations. Both are sticky and insoluble in water or oil, but the 90 percent type is ground and more convenient to use. I always grind the dark brown powder along with some oatmeal (not instant) in the coffee grinder for a finer particle size and a less sticky material. Add ground propolis at the trace as an exfoliant and for colored specks of texture.

## Q: *How does borax affect a bar of soap?*

A: I am not sure. Borax — sodium borate — is a white crystalline mineral used as an emulsifier, a cleanser, a preservative, a texturizer, and a water softener. I use a cosmetic-grade borax in my creams as an emulsifier — an ingredient that binds together the oil and water portions.

I have yet to determine borax's effect on a cold-process soap. Whether I include or exclude it, my final bars seem to vary little. Some soapmakers feel that borax acts as a gentle cleanser and opens pores. Since all of the ones whom I've talked to use a laundry-grade borax found in the supermarket, I suspect that it is not gentle. I don't know whether or not it opens pores. The one interesting possibility is that it may speed the sudsing action of the soap. Lather, of course, is only as generous as the amount of smaller-chain fatty-acid oils such as coconut or palm kernel, but borax may cause soap to release its lather more quickly. It may be that my mind is tricking me, but I think I've noticed this one benefit of borax. To give borax a try, add about 2 tablespoons (30 ml) per 12 ounces (340.2 g) of sodium hydroxide to the freshly made lye solution. Use a cosmetic grade.

Borax ◀ ·······································

## Q: *Is it necessary to test the pH of soap?*

A: I rarely test the lather of soap for its pH because all of my superfatted bars are gentle, though still slightly alkaline. The goal is not to make a neutral bar, but instead to keep the pH within a range of 5.5 to 10. It is thought that the skin can adjust to a pH of 10.5 more easily than it can to the synthetic chemicals that are added to commercial soap to lower pH. Advertisers have successfully turned pH into a phenomenon, but my hands-on experimentation reveals little to no difference in the skin's reaction to a pH of 7 versus a pH of 10 (of course, more extreme values do make a difference). Inspect soap for any visual oddities that may reveal excess or poorly blended lye, and be sure that

pH ◀ ·······································

soap is moisturizing and not drying, but don't worry about pH unless your practical application suggests a problem.

And remember that it is probably best to think of pH in terms of a safe range rather than one particular safe value.

*Stearic acid*

Q: *Should I add stearic acid for harder bars?*

A: Stearic acid is a saturated fatty acid, usually derived from either beef tallow or hog fat, though a vegetable form is available from palm oil. Stearic acid is separated from the neutral fat by reacting the neutral oil with a strong base. Within industry, fatty acids are split from the glycerol portion of a triglyceride; this pure fatty acid is then combined with an alkali to make soap. Emollients are added to these formulas to compensate for the loss of the glycerin.

Those triglycerides with high percentages of saturated fatty acids produce the hardest bars of soap, and some soapmakers include them in their formulas to contribute hardness to the final bars. The particular fatty acids used determine physical properties such as lather and hardness, and stearic acid makes hard bars with long-lasting, thin lathers. But straight stearic acid makes soap very hard — too hard. Without the glycerol portion of its triglyceride, and without some percentage of unsaturated fatty acids, the soap made from pure stearic acid is hard and brittle. Some cold-process soapmakers thus add a small amount of stearic acid to their neutral oil formulas to compensate for the percentage of unsaturated oil in the blend.

Though it shouldn't be used without other less saturated oils or fatty acids, stearic acid can be incorporated into a well-balanced soap formula to contribute texture. Keep in mind that straight stearic acid can be an allergen for some people, so carefully create its formulas to include emollient materials. Without the glycerol, pure stearic acid has a saponification value of 197; treat this fatty acid as just another "fat or oil" when calculating SAP value (see chapter 13, pages 245–247). Melt the stearic acid along with the other solid fats and oils, adding approximately 1 tablespoon (15 ml) of stearic acid per 1 pound (453.6 g) of total fats and oils.

I do not incorporate stearic acid into my soap formulas. I have no need for it. My philosophy is "less is more," and I only include an ingredient if its contribution is meaningful. A well-balanced soap formula will produce very hard bars once they have cured. Only after solid service will the remaining sliver of soap give way. All soaps, including tallow soaps and synthetic soaps, become soft toward the end of their usefulness. Since my soap is hard and long-lasting, I feel no need to change a perfectly simple blend for the sake of a very slight improvement.

Though I choose to use only the neutral fats and oils, many soapmakers are pleased with what the addition of stearic acid contributes to their soaps. It gets more stubborn batches going and it produces very hard bars of soap. Ask Henkel Corporation for a local distributor of its vegetable stearic acid (see "Suppliers" in the appendix).

## Q: Are fixatives necessary?

A: Fixatives are chemicals that reduce the tendency of a scent to vaporize, making it last longer. Certain plant materials — roots, leaves, peel, essential oil, and resin — blend with certain essential oils and "hold" them steady for longer than they would last on their own. A synergy strengthens the scent and protects it from quickly evaporating.

Other than the coincidental benefits I receive from having chosen essential oils that happen to "fix" one another, I do not incorporate fixatives into my soap formulas. A well-balanced formula — one with complementary fats, oils, nutrients, and essential oils, and the correct ratio of fats and oils to water to sodium hydroxide — will retain its scent for two to three years and longer. Since I don't include any ingredient that does not contribute something meaningful to my soap, I leave out fixatives.

If a scent is disappearing quickly, it is probably due to an inferior oil. Some soapmakers complain about citrus blends losing their scent quickly, but I've not had this problem, and I attribute this to the fine-quality essential oils I use. The cost of good fixatives is probably higher than that of purchasing the good essential oils in the first place.

Common scent fixatives:

♦ Balsam of Peru (may cause contact dermatitis)
♦ Benzoin gum (styrax benzoin — may cause allergic reactions)
♦ Cedarwood chips or oil
♦ Clary sage
♦ Cloves
♦ Lemon peel
♦ Orange peel
♦ Orris root
♦ Patchouli leaves and oil (may irritate some)
♦ Sandalwood (may irritate some)
♦ Storax oil
♦ Tangerine peel
♦ Vetiver

# Q: *What is rebatching?*

A: Rebatching is the cold-process soapmaker's attempt to create a milled bar of soap. In theory this is a great idea, but I've not yet used a rebatched soap that could compare favorably to a milled soap.

The virtues of a milled soap are that it can be made rock hard and silky smooth, and that it requires less essential oil for a strong scent. In milling, fresh soap is flattened paper-thin between sets of rollers, then shredded into flakes. Once shredded, it is much less alkaline than fresh soap, and scent is added to the flakes before they are squeezed and protruded through extrusion machinery. The soap flakes tightly compact and are no longer distinguishable within the resulting dense bars of soap.

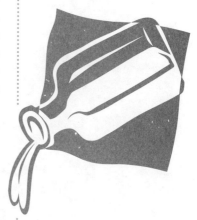

The continuous compression of the soap flakes, combined with some synthetic materials used just for this purpose, create hard, polished bars of soap. Milled soap formulas also contain synthetic substances that make the soap flakes less sticky and more plastic, to prevent them from sticking to the large metal rollers.

A cold-process vegetable soap contains too much natural glycerin to accommodate milling machinery, and the physical attributes of the milled soap have yet to be duplicated by rebatching. To rebatch is to make a batch of cold-process soap, let it cure for a few days or longer, melt it down slowly over a double boiler and very low heat with little or no water, let the melted soap cool just enough to thicken, and, finally, scent the soap and pour it into molds. The goals are to achieve harder bars and to use less scent, since the supposedly less alkaline soap (after a short cure) will not "eat" so much of the essential oils.

Try rebatching for the sake of experimentation; I personally feel that it's more fuss than it's worth. Without the milling machinery (which won't work without a milling formula), rebatched soap cannot be compacted tightly enough to achieve the gloss and the hardness of milled soap. It can look grainy and patched together. Cold-process soap takes longer than a few days to become mild enough to be impervious to scent, so wait a few weeks before you shred the soap, instead of just a few days, or the benefit of using less scent will not be a meaningful one.

Also keep in mind that a true milled soap is completely dry before it is pressed through the series of rollers. In designing my laundry soap, I learned firsthand that when soaked in water, shredded sodium soap often becomes gelatinous. The home version of milling soap — rebatching — is likely to produce varied results, depending upon the composition of the soap base, processing temperatures, and environmental conditions. Too many factors determine the texture of the final rebatched soap for the soapmaker to feel confident that success can be reliably achieved.

Adding fruits and vegetables ⋯⋯⋯⋯⋯⋯⋯⟶

## Q: *Should fruits and vegetables be included in soap?*

A: Though most cosmetic ingredients are not edible, some are food-grade, such as the fats and oils, herbs, cornmeal, oatmeal, milk, and honey that are incorporated into soap formulas. Some soapmakers add fresh fruits and vegetables to their formulas; they make soap with strawberries, cucumbers, carrots, avocados, kiwis, or lettuce. These items are thought to add emollience and cleansing power.

I add biodegradable ingredients only if they contribute meaningfully to my final bars of soap. Excess vegetable fats and oils (beyond what is needed for saponification), chlorophyll, fresh aloe vera gel, and honey break down even within carefully formulated, superfatted soap. I appreciate the year or so of freshness that such bars give me and ask no more from them. I choose this more vulnerable formulation over a fully saponified bar that can last for centuries.

Some soapmakers do not need even a year from a soap; they make soap in small quantities and use it within two to six months. These soapmakers can include food in their soap formulas.

After evaluating the needs that a particular soap should satisfy, you can determine what ingredients to include. If emollience and cleansing take precedence over shelf life (though at least a year is hoped for), then you can include some organic materials, though only a carefully calculated percentage. If shelf life is your determining factor, you will want a more fully saponified soap and have to sacrifice some degree of skin-care benefit. If shelf life is irrelevant to you and emollience and personality are key, then by all means empty the produce compartment of your refrigerator into the soap pan, and have fun!

## Q: *What is tea tree oil?*

Tea tree oil

A: The many species of Melaleuca trees are native to Australia, and one in particular, *Melaleuca alternifolia,* has been used medicinally since the aboriginal people discovered its germicidal qualities. As a group of species, Melaleuca trees have been known as tea trees since the time when their leaves were first used to prepare an herbal tea.

The essential oil from the *Melaleuca alternifolia* is used to treat a wide range of skin disorders, as it is thought to affect fungi, viruses, and bacteria. Tea tree oil is used to treat acne, sunburn, dandruff, burns, oily skin, rashes, insect bites, cuts, and infected wounds. It is quickly absorbed by the skin and thought to speed healing.

Though it is used in its concentrated form to treat burns and acne, some experts believe that tea tree oil should be diluted for most skin-care treatment. It is also advisable to avoid eye contact. Whenever I use tea tree oil as a nutrient and an essential oil in soap, I blend it with other pure essential oils, using about ½ ounce (14 g) of tea tree oil per 1 pound (453.6 g) of fats. Add the tea tree oil blend just before you pour the soap. Most of the people in my life dislike its strong medicinal scent, but I love it, especially in a blend.

## Q: *How does beeswax affect a soap formula?*

Beeswax

A: Some soapmakers include beeswax in their formulas for the hardness it contributes to the final bars. The smell of honey is a bonus. Along with borax, beeswax holds fatty oils in an emulsion within moisturizing creams and lotions.

Plant extracts

Beeswax is obtained from the honeycomb of honeybees. As worker bees consume large quantities of honey, a waxy substance secreted by their wax glands forms on their bodies. Using this wax, they build cells to accommodate their eggs and honey. This arrangement of cells is called a honeycomb. Once processors extract the honey from the honeycomb, they melt the honeycomb in boiling water, and the wax that rises to the surface is collected and filtered. This is the wax that can be used in soap. More commonly, beeswax is used in candles, lubricants, cosmetics, polishes, and chewing gum.

Beeswax is an ester, a compound formed by the reaction of an acid and an alcohol. A triglyceride is three fatty acids attached to glycerol — an alcohol with three hydroxyl (OH) groups; beeswax is primarily palmitic acid (a saturated fatty acid) attached to a monohydroxy alcohol (an alcohol with one hydroxyl group).

Fats and oil and beeswax are all esters, meaning that they all can be saponified. Therefore, beeswax is melted along with the other saturated fats at the beginning of the soapmaking process. Because beeswax has a higher melting point, you will need slightly higher soapmaking temperatures (around 100°F [38°C]). Many soapmakers love the rock-hard beeswax soaps, but try to keep the percentage of beeswax in a formula to around 1.5 percent of the total fats and oils (¼ ounce [7 g] of beeswax per 1 pound [453.6 g] of fat). Too much beeswax makes the bars sticky and gummy, and inhibits lathering.

Natural beeswax is dark yellow and has a honeylike scent. White beeswax, which has been bleached, is yellowish white and can cause dermatitis upon contact. Note that some people have a sensitivity to beeswax products and that vegans will not use any bee by-products.

Q: *What are the differences among an essential oil, a concrete, and an absolute?*

A: All three of these are highly concentrated substances derived from plants, and they carry the plants' scents and beneficial properties. They are extracted from leaves, bark, flowers, roots, and fruit, though different extraction processes retrieve slightly different concentrations of material. They differ most with respect to physical state: Essential oils are almost always liquid; concretes are solid or semisolid; and absolutes are liquid or semisolid.

An essential oil is the volatile (quick to evaporate) oil obtained from the odorous parts of one particular plant. Inside the plant, the oil defends against predators and disease, and attracts beneficial insects. It is extracted through distillation or expression, and though some are semisolid, most are in liquid form.

The solid fraction of a plant's scented parts is extracted using hydrocarbon solvents; the liquid portion is left behind, and this solid or semisolid residue is called a concrete. Concretes are used to make perfumes, but they are difficult to incorporate into soaps and other mediums due to their low solubility. Often, they are converted into absolutes, which are easier to work with.

Absolutes are extracted from concretes using alcohol. The resulting liquid or semisolid is thick and slow-flowing, though more soluble than concretes.

Q: *How does cassia oil differ from cinnamon oil?*

A: Cassia oil and cinnamon oil are both casually referred to as cinnamon oil, though they are obtained from two different cinnamon trees (of related species) and produce very different cinnamon powders and oils. Both oils are antimicrobial, astringent, and antiseptic (but see the warning, at right).

Cassia oil is derived from the leaves and twigs of the cassia cinnamon tree of China *(Cinnamomum cassia)*. Its scent is strong, but not as sweet and delicate as that of cinnamon bark oil. Cassia oil is more affordable, though, and produces a nice cinnamon scent in soap. Cassia bark is used to make the baking and cooking spice cinnamon.

Cinnamon bark oil and cinnamon leaf oil are derived from the Ceylon cinnamon tree *(Cinnamomum zeylanicum)*. The leaf oil is far less expensive than the bark oil, and also less expensive than cassia oil. Its flavor is hot, spicy, and bitter — more like cloves than true

**WARNING**

Though I have safely blended cassia oil with other pure essential oils, cassia oil and cinnamon bark oil contain large quantities of cinnamic aldehyde, which can be toxic to skin.

cinnamon. Cinnamon bark oil is very expensive — overkill for the soapmaker — but it has the warmest, sweetest flavor.

Soap names ·················································➤

Q: *What are the meanings of sodium palmitate, sodium stearate, sodium tallowate, and so on, found as ingredients on soap labels?*

A: Each is a fancy way of saying soap. Each is the sodium soap of a particular fat or oil. Sodium tallowate is the sodium salt (or soap) produced when tallow is reacted with lye. Sodium stearate is saponified stearic acid — soap produced by reacting stearic acid with lye. Sodium palmitate is saponified palm oil. Many companies have no desire to list on their labels sodium hydroxide or tallow or stearic acid (they are afraid of scaring consumers away). So in a day when many soaps are unaffected by cosmetic labeling laws, companies creatively find precise, technical words to describe their final products, instead of listing the ingredients in plain language.

Soapmaking
in the Library

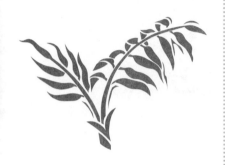

# PART 2

# CHAPTER 10
## Resins

Trees have been tapped since the beginning of time for their therapeutic resins, and there is something comforting and sustaining about the continual flow of life from these ancient friends. Primitive civilizations relied upon the medicinal value of resins to treat a variety of disorders. Today, they are still used for their antiseptic, antioxidant, and preservative qualities. Soapmakers are eager to incorporate resins into soap because of their medicinal value, vanillalike scent and rich, brown tones.

Unfortunately, resins are not compatible with cold-process soapmaking. They are semisolid and have the consistency of thick, sticky tar. They are soluble in alcohol but not at all in water or fatty acids. I have mashed and ground quantities of resins into the minimum amount of alcohol required for solubility, and I have successfully added this resin/alcohol mixture before the trace, but this process is a nuisance, and not worth the effort. After my experiments, though I liked the soap, I decided that the fit was not a comfortable one, and that I was forcing the issue. Resins are better used in other applications.

The better news is that resins can be incorporated into transparent soap formulas for darker transparency, since alcohol is a major ingredient in these formulas. The best news for the cold-process soapmaker is that an essential oil that strongly resembles a particular resin in character and scent is distilled from the resin, and can be added to soap just like any other essential oil. A few have wonderful vanillalike scents, some smell of pine, and others are offensive.

## Incorporating Resins into Soap

I know of some soapmakers who use both the resins and their oils for the maximum effect. The medicinal benefits and unusual scents cause them to push this square peg into a round hole. Since a cold-process soap does not accept the resin in any phase — lye, oils, or final soap mixture — you must try to sneak it in. Cold-process soap seizes from the addition of too much alcohol, so dissolve the resin in the smallest amount of alcohol possible and add it at the trace along with your other essential oils. Pour the soap into molds as quickly as possible; it will begin to solidify in your soapmaking pan if you are not swift enough. Resins should account for no more than .1 percent of your soapmaking ingredients.

## KINDS OF RESINS

The term *resin* refers to several kinds, including oleoresins, balsams, gums, and rosin. The distinction among these kinds of resins is blurred, and often the terms are used interchangeably. But each resin is slightly different.

All resins are vegetable secretions found in trees and shrubs — mixtures of fatty acids and essential oils. They are compounds of carbon, hydrogen, and small amounts of oxygen; they are hard when cool, sticky when warm. Natural resins can be divided into three main categories: saplike mixtures that flow from plants; those extracted from wood by solvents; and fossil resins found with the preserved remains of animals and plants. Most resins are oleoresins from tree saps.

The consistencies of the different resins vary. The ones with little volatile oil are hard resins. Some resins, after being extracted from the plant, are dissolved into volatile oils and become semisolids. Others are combined with gums in the form of gum resins.

### Oleoresins

Some resins are found in combination with fragrant essential oils; these are called oleoresins. Oleoresins are secreted by the pine family within a complex network of canals in the sapwood and inner bark of the trees. They protect the trees from disease and moisture loss by serving as a barrier. Once the oleoresin is exposed to air, the volatile oil in the oleoresin evaporates and leaves behind a hard, shiny resin that seals off the trees. Oleoresins are obtained from wounds into the bark. Most types are

**FOSSIL RESIN**

Amber, one of the fossil resins, is a hard, yellowish brown, translucent substance formed from the resins of extinct pine trees. Perhaps millions of years ago, this resinous material combined with the oils in the trees, and when the oils reacted with oxygen, hard resins formed. Over time, the pine trees became buried under water or under the ground, and the hard resins developed into pieces of amber.

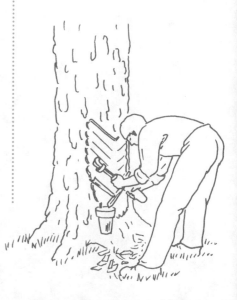

Oleoresins are extracted from trees in the pine family.

semisolid and sticky at room temperature, but become soft and stickier at higher temperatures.

Turpentine is one oleoresin; it is obtained from conifers, such as pine and fir trees. Benzoin is another oleoresin, also known as styrax benzoin. It is obtained by cutting notches into the bark of the styrax tree of Southeast Asia. It is used medicinally to treat cuts and dry, irritated skin, and is an antioxidant, antiseptic, styptic, deodorant, and astringent. I've read about the sweet, balsamic scent of benzoin, but I must have sampled another type. There was nothing vanillalike about it; it reminded me of ether.

## Balsam

Balsams, such as copaiba, tolu, and Peru, are spicy-smelling resinous mixtures obtained from evergreen trees. Their compositions vary, but often contain oleoresins and terpenes — such as benzoic acid, cinnamic acid, benzoates, and cinnamates. They are soluble in organic liquids, such as alcohol, but insoluble in water, and they are incapable of saponification.

Balsam of tolu is a pleasant-smelling, reddish brown substance obtained from a South American tree, *Myroxylon toluiferum.* It is used as an antiseptic, a fixative, and a soft, hyacinthlike fragrance in soap and cosmetics. Though listed as a possible allergen, tolu balsam is used to treat dry, chapped skin and skin wounds.

Balsam of Peru is found in the tree *Myroxylon peruiferum,* which grows in dense forests near the coast in El Salvador. Peru balsam is a dark brown liquid with a lingering vanilla scent due to its vanillin content; it offers soap this pleasant smell along with a creamy lather. It is soothing, astringent, and mildly antiseptic, and has been used to treat skin irritations, though be aware that it has also been known to irritate the skin and cause dermatitis for some people. The oil also carries the deep vanilla scent of the balsam.

Storax — sometimes called styrax, sweet oriental gum, or gum storax — is found in the inner bark of the *Liquidambar styraciflora* tree. Storax is a semiliquid substance, usually brown or gray. It is used to treat skin wounds, and considered anti-inflammatory, antimicrobial, and antiseptic, though it can irritate some people. Storax is also used as a fixative and a preservative in soaps and cosmetics. The scent of storax is often described using such adjectives as *sweet, balsamic,* and *slightly spicy;* I must be missing something, because again I detect only an unpleasant smell that reminds me of ether.

Copaiba balsam is tapped from the trunk of the *Copaifera landsdorfi* tree. For centuries it has been used medicinally by the native people in the Amazon rain forest to heal, soothe, and soften skin. It is thought to be bacteriostatic and disinfectant. Copaiba oil is obtained from the balsam for use as a fixative in scenting soap and cosmetics. The resin has the sticky, semisolid consistency of other resins and must be incorporated as such, but copaiba oil is added to the soap at the trace along with other pure essential oils.

## Gum Resin

Gum resin contains natural gum, oil, and coloring matter. A sticky, polysaccharide substance, gum resin is gelatinous when moist, hard when dry, and water-soluble. It is found in the leaves, bark, and roots of the various plants that secrete this resin. Essential oils are distilled from gum resins and contribute many of the same properties that the resins do.

Gum benzoin, one kind of gum, has a warm, wonderful scent. It is an antioxidant, an antiseptic, and an anti-inflammatory. Though gum benzoin is often used to heal chapped, dry skin and other skin disorders, it is an allergen for some people. As a perfume, it blends nicely with frankincense, rose, sandalwood, cloves, and juniper berry. Gum benzoin is often confused with storax, one of the balsam resins. This is because storax is also called styrax, and gum benzoin is obtained from the botanical source *Styrax benzoin.*

Myrrh and frankincense are other gum resins used as astringents, antiseptics, and anti-inflammatories. Myrrh also has antimicrobial properties. Both are thought to be nonirritating and are used to perfume soap and cosmetics. To incorporate these resins in a powdered form look for ground myrrh and frankincense (but do not expect medicinal value).

## Rosin

Rosin is a hard, translucent resin obtained from oleoresin, tall oil (a by-product of the wood pulp industry), or the dead stumps of pine trees. It is available in the form of gum rosin, wood rosin, and tall oil rosin. Once the essential oils are distilled from the oleoresin, the rosin is left behind. Primarily, rosin is used industrially in sizing paper, making linoleum, and making varnishes and paints.

Rosin was used for many years in the manufacture of lower-grade soap, contributing lather to opaque formulas and transparency to transparent and translucent formulas. Most varieties make darker, softer soap. Rosin is thought to increase lathering, but I was skeptical that it would do so meaningfully until recently, when I included it in an opaque formula. Only 4 ounces (113.4 g) of rosin added to a 5-pound (2.3-kg) batch of soap produced the quickest, fluffiest lather I had ever seen, to my surprise. I used gum rosin, which did not darken the soap, though the bars did take longer to harden.

Include some cocoa butter or beeswax, and apply only a 5 to 10 percent sodium hydroxide discount. This glasslike resin is insoluble in all soapmaking phases at lower temperatures, but it does melt at higher temperatures. Heat the rosin along with the solid fats to 180°F (82.2°C) to completely melt it; then add the liquid oils and cool the mixture to 100°F (38°C). The lye solution is added to the fats and oils at 90°F (32°C). Cold-process rosin soap can be slightly grainy, so be sure to beat the mixture well. Note that rosin can cause contact dermatitis in sensitive individuals.

# CHAPTER 11
## Minerals and Clays

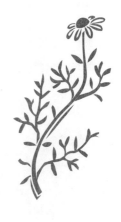

A variety of minerals and clays are added to skin-care products for their color, texture, and absorbency. Clays (combinations of finely ground minerals) are also thought to help the skin function more normally by clearing the pores of excess sebum, toxins, and dirt. A clear path with no blockages enables the skin to "clean house" on its own, absorbing required moisture from the air and releasing impurities and excess oils, which can then be washed away. Clay and water are blended into a slurry and spread on the skin to dry; the resulting "pack" is astringent and cleansing. This treatment is an ancient one, but in question are both its relevance to the soapmaker and the purity of its raw materials. It is unclear how effectively minerals and clays work within a bar of soap, and purity seems to differ from mine to mine.

There is not enough data to definitively declare these materials safe or unsafe, helpful or useless, within skin-care products. Many natural-cosmetic companies include clays and minerals in their products and appear to be doing so without incident. Customers rave about the results. But some of these materials crop up on lists of hazardous substances, usually cited for mild to moderate skin-related problems. This may be another case of small quantities doing no harm (but how much good, in that case?).

Some elements, such as gold and silver, are found in nature in a pure state, but most materials obtained from the earth are found as compounds or mixtures along with other less desirable substances. Clays contain minerals, and minerals are often found in mixtures of clay. Understanding the differences between minerals and clays is important for soapmakers. Beginning soapmakers are likely to believe a supplier who confidently explains that ultramarine is a natural mineral and that rose ocher is a clay. I know this from personal experience. In time I learned that the ultramarine used to color soap is not a natural mineral and that rose ocher does not exist. Though precise definitions distinguish clays from minerals, they are generally lumped together and referred to broadly as inorganic minerals, because they all share similar chemical and physical traits. A clearer understanding of the distinctions permits the soapmaker to choose ingredients more selectively.

All of the minerals discussed in this chapter fall under the general heading of inorganic minerals. Iron oxide, titanium dioxide, ochers, clays, ultramarine, and pearlescent pigments all contain minerals. Though it is impossible to disassociate one material from another (with so much in common), for purposes of organization I have divided them into two main categories: minerals — including red iron oxide, black iron oxide, titanium dioxide, ultramarine, and pearlescent pigments; and clays — including montmorillonite, kaolin, and ochers.

## MINERALS

The term *mineral* is often loosely applied to include all nonliving (inorganic) portions of the earth's crust. This overly broad definition would include such true minerals as gold, silver, salt, gypsum, talc, ochers, oxides, and pencil lead, but would also include coal, natural gas, petroleum, and sand — none of which is technically a mineral.

Though a few minerals are found in nature as pure chemical elements, most are chemical compounds. A narrower definition limits the term *mineral* to those elements or compounds found in the form of crystals that are created by inorganic processes of nature. They may be found as individual crystals, or within mixtures of various minerals and rocks. They are usually formed in one or more of the following ways: as precipitation from liquids, such as oceans, hot springs, or geysers; from molten rock (the cooling and hardening of magma); or from solid rock that undergoes a change to a more crystalline structure when affected by heat, pressure, and water.

### WARNING

I *do not discuss the full range of artists' pigments in this book, because I warn against their use as soap colorants. Many pigments, such as carbon black, raw sienna, zinc white, manganese violet, mars yellow, and chromium green, are thought to be inert materials, but I am skeptical. Chromium and carbon are suspected to be carcinogenic when inhaled, and many artists' minerals are toxic in powdered form. Note that these pigments are also likely to contain impurities.*

Technically, a mineral satisfies the following four requirements:

◆ It is naturally occurring.
◆ It is composed of materials that were never alive.
◆ Its chemical and molecular formulas are the same wherever
  it is found.
◆ The atoms within it are arranged in a predictable, regular pattern
  and form solid crystals.

For example, red iron oxide, or ferric oxide, which is a mineral, has a chemical formula of $Fe_2O_3$ whether it is found in Norway, Brazil, or the United States. But the calcium found in milk is not a mineral, since it does not have a crystalline structure. Nor are organic materials such as coal and oil minerals, because they were once living, and because they do not have definite chemical formulas.

Minerals are not organized according to the elements they have in common. Instead, they are classified with respect to chemical composition and crystalline form. Oxides belong to one group of mineral classifications. Iron oxides and titanium dioxide are the ones most relevant to the soapmaker because they cure the minerals more commonly used to color cosmetics and soap (not my recommendation).

## Iron Oxides

Iron oxides are combinations of iron and oxygen. Iron is rarely found in its natural state, and instead exists in compounds with oxygen, carbon, sulfur, and hydrogen in the form of ores. Three combinations of iron and oxygen, in particular, interest the soapmaker: $Fe_2O_3$ (red iron oxide) and $Fe_3O_4$ (black iron oxide).

Some soapmakers incorporate iron oxides into their soaps, often in the form of synthetically produced iron oxide. Most of the iron oxide available is synthetic, due to FDA regulations that strictly prohibit the use of natural iron oxide in cosmetics. The issue is purity, and natural iron oxides are more likely than the synthetic versions to contain high levels of impurities. Note that many soaps are exempt from this regulation, though, since they are not technically defined as cosmetics (see chapter 17, page 270).

## Natural Red Iron Oxide

Natural red iron oxide, also known as hematite, is mined from deposits. Most samples are polluted with frighteningly high levels of heavy metals and other impurities, such as nickel and chromium. For this reason, the FDA has not preapproved natural iron oxide for use as a cosmetic colorant. And while a loophole may exist enabling the soapmaker to use natural iron oxide as a colorant, consider the intent behind the FDA's restriction. Though it may not legally apply to soapmaking, it is cause for concern. Some deposits contain fewer impurities than others, and some companies do a better job than others removing the contaminants, but it is difficult for the soapmaker to determine these levels in an unapproved product, short of testing each purchase. One expert at the FDA has yet to obtain a safe iron oxide sample from nature after twenty years of research.

## Red Hematite

Another red iron oxide is made from ocher — a natural mixture of earth and iron compounds (see the following section on clays). The primary difference between red iron oxide and ocher relates to water. Ocher, known as goethite, is actually hydrated iron — iron oxide chemically bound to water — and red hematite is iron oxide without the water. When ocher is heated beyond 212°F (100°C), the chemically bound water is driven from it, converting yellow ocher (hydrated iron oxide) into red hematite (iron oxide without chemically bound water). The structures of the crystals in the ocher change form, producing a near replica of natural red iron oxide.

*Red iron oxide* and *hematite* are chemical terms, and *ocher* is a geological term. Red iron oxide answers to all three names, but technically,

**SOAPMAKING NOTE**

Oxides can be mixed to achieve lighter and darker shades. Red iron oxide can be mixed with titanium dioxide (see entry) to lighten its brick color to a shade of rose.

once ocher becomes calcined (heated and converted to red hematite), it is from then on known as hematite.

### Synthetic Red Iron Oxide

Synthetic red iron oxide is made from recycled scrap iron and recaptured sulfur from fossil fuels — converting these wastes into usable pigment. Machine shop turnings, free of metals that could cause contamination, are dissolved in sulfuric acid, after which the sulfuric acid is recovered. Further sulfuric-acid treatment creates ferric sulfate, which, after more reactions, decomposes into red iron oxide. The size and the shape of the crystals (red iron oxides are spherical) determine the predominant wavelengths reflected by the crystals (the colors our eyes see): Small spheres reflect reds and yellows, with more yellow and less blue; larger spheres reflect reds, with some blue and purple-maroon.

### Synthetic Black Iron Oxide

Black iron oxide, known as magnetite, is found in small amounts in red iron oxide and exists independently in nature, but is almost always produced synthetically. Its crystals are not uniform, and grinding them breaks the crystalline structure and changes the absorption of color from black to brown. The synthetic version is produced much as synthetic red iron oxide is — though different chemicals are used — and its crystalline structure is cubic instead of spherical. The structure is responsible for the black color; it keeps light from escaping by absorbing much of it and reflecting very little.

### Titanium Dioxide

Titanium dioxide is a metal oxide used as an approved white coloring agent in cosmetics. It also produces an opaque effect, making its products unaffected by light. Titanium dioxide is most commonly used in foundation makeup, face and bath powder, eye shadow, lipstick, and sunscreen.

**CAUTION**

Both the synthetic and the natural forms of iron oxide may cause skin irritation, along with burns and inflammation of the eyelids. Some people have no obvious reaction, but others are more vulnerable. I do not recommend using iron oxides as soap colorants.

Soapmakers add titanium dioxide to cold-process soap at trace as a bright white colorant, or to a marbled white portion against the linen-white base. Though many natural-cosmetic companies seem to use it safely, some studies suggest that it may cause skin irritation, along with redness, tearing, and irritation of the eyes. Most studies find no toxicity for external application, but warn of lung damage from inhalation. Titanium dioxide is available in both natural and synthetic forms. If you want the natural version, be sure to ask for it specifically.

## Ultramarines

There was a day when ultramarine pigment was derived from the gem lapis lazuli, but this expensive stone is no longer the source of the brilliant blue color. The Egyptians and Romans called lapis lazuli "sapphire," and mixed the ground mineral with milk to treat boils and ulcers. But today's ultramarines are sodium aluminum sulfur silicates made synthetically by heating a mixture of kaolin, sodium carbonate, sulfur, silica, carbon, and resin to very high temperatures. Ultramarine blue, pink, and violet are chemically and structurally almost identical; only a slight difference in ratios of atoms accounts for the three very different, vibrant colors. They are all approved colorants for external use; the soapmaker can easily obtain beautiful shades using these synthetic pigments.

The blue form of ultramarine is made industrially in very hot ovens. First, the above mixture is heated to 1472°F (800°C), after which it is cooled to around 752°F (400°C). Then, when the oven door is cracked open slightly, the blue color starts to develop.

This blue ultramarine is the base of the other two colors. As blue ultramarine cools to around 752°F (400°C), oxidation takes place. At around 392°F (200°C), ammonium chloride is added; some of the sodium ions react with the ammonium chloride, and these sodium ions are replaced with hydrogen ions. The result is a violet ultramarine. Finally, continuing this process using the violet ultramarine as the base produces pink ultramarine, which contains even more sodium ions than the other two forms. Once color is achieved, the pigments are washed and eventually ground to the desired particle size.

Generally, synthetic ultramarine is thought to be nontoxic. But as in the cases of so many other questionable materials, natural and synthetic, the studies have not been exactly on point for the soapmaker (though even many "natural" soapmakers seem to use ultramarines safely). The more general studies suggest that synthetic ultramarines are inert and safe to use within skin-care products. Since only 1 teaspoon (5 ml) of ultramarine blue (or 3–4 teaspoons of violet and pink) is needed to color 5 pounds (2.3 kg) of soap, there is only a small amount of colorant in each bar. Still, quantity is not always a reliable gauge, so exercise the same caution that you would for any questionable natural colorant.

## Pearlescent Pigments

Some soapmakers use pearlescent pigments to add sparkles to their soap. These pigments are created in the lab by coating microscopic, transparent slices of mica with iron oxides or titanium dioxide and arranging them in parallel layers. Through the layers light is absorbed and reflected, creating flashes of glitter and pearls called pearlescence. Brighter colors are created by adding synthetic colorants to the pearlescent pigment formulations.

Pearlescent pigments are synthetic, because natural forms of iron oxide and titanium dioxide do not adhere to the mica, and because FDA regulations restrict the use of pure oxides within cosmetics (see "Iron Oxides," above).

Different colors of transparent glitter are achieved by varying the thickness of the titanium dioxide and iron oxide layers that coat the mica. Iron oxide reflects deeper bronze colors, while titanium dioxide reflects brighter earth colors. Gold sparkles are created by superthin layers of titanium dioxide, which emit gold-colored interference.

## CLAYS

Within the earth, hot magma melts and flows toward the earth's surface but is obstructed thousands of feet underground, where it remains for long periods of time. As it very slowly cools, it is exposed to hot internal gases such as boron, fluorine, carbon dioxide, and water, which over time contribute to the breakdown of the magma into clay. If the magma reaches the surface of the earth through volcanic eruptions, it cools quickly and forms fine-grained rocks that are not valuable. But with very slow cooling periods, large crystals form during a complex series of chemical reactions. The cooling magma crystallizes in different stages into varying minerals; granite is the last rock to crystallize. As a category, the resulting rock is called igneous rock.

Clays are fine-grained particles that originated thousands of years ago as igneous rock (hot molten rock from the interior of the earth) or metamorphic rock (rock that changed form due to the heat and pressure of igneous reactions nearby). Few clays are found where they originated (primary clay). Most are transported by water and ice to other areas (sedimentary clay). Over thousands of years of freezing and thawing, the rock disintegrates and washes away. Further weathering breaks already decomposed pieces into smaller and finer particles.

Due to all of its travel and interaction, clay is rarely found in nature as only one kind; instead, it is usually mixed with other clays. All clays are combinations of fine-grained earthy materials and finely ground minerals in the form of small crystals. They are perhaps the finest-grained materials obtained from the earth. Clays, water, air, and organic matter are the four major portions of the soil.

Chemically, clays are silicates — compounds of silicon, oxygen, and one or more metals (often aluminum) that are chemically combined with water. Approximately 30 percent of all minerals occur in the form of silicates. The silicates are arranged in layers, or sheets, with water trapped between. Clays are known for their ability to expand, since they can absorb large quantities of water between their stacked silicate sheets.

## Clays and Skin Care

Both kaolin and montmorillonite (some companies refer to it as bentonite or French green clay) are used by natural-cosmetic companies within their masks, soaps, and powders. How effective clay is within a

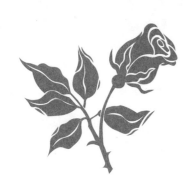

soap is unclear, but perhaps it does have astringent and cleansing properties. Many people claim this to be so, and I suspect that they might be right, since I find clay soaps to be slightly drying. Clays may be best suited to people with oily complexions.

Kaolin is generally gentler and purer than montmorillonite, though many soapmakers feel comfortable using them interchangeably. Kaolin is white, montmorillonite often gray-green. Red or rose clays are often not true montmorillonite, as they are usually produced industrially by combining genuine montmorillonite with high percentages of iron oxide.

## Kaolin

Different combinations of rocks create different clays. The purest clay is kaolin, obtained from granite that was once melted rock, or magma. It is composed principally of the mineral kaolinite, with few impurities. Other rocks form clays that are less pure. They often contain different kinds of rock — usually a combination of molten rock and the surrounding hard rock in the earth, called country rock. This country rock is dramatically altered by the heat and pressure of the surrounding hot magma, and by chemically reacting with magma and trapped gases. The resulting clays contain more elements and more complex compounds than kaolin does, and are therefore not as pure as this granite-derived clay.

## Montmorillonite

Some materials, such as mica and montmorillonite, are found in clays but are not technically clays themselves. Mica is more like sand and affects the texture of a clay. *Montmorillonite* has two definitions: It is the classification heading for all clay minerals that have absorbing, expanding structures; and it is also the name of a specific, finely ground mineral within that classification that contributes strength and plasticity to its mixtures.

The absorbent material bentonite is one of the montmorillonite minerals. It is composed principally of the mineral montmorillonite, and both are so claylike that they are commonly referred to as clays, though technically they are minerals, not clays. While bentonite is found in small quantities within various clays, it is found on its own as a by-product of the decomposition of volcanic ash.

## Ochers

Ochers are mixtures of sand, clay, and iron compounds (such as iron oxides) that derive their color from the iron oxide. They are considered more clays than minerals. Yellow and brown types are obtained from different layers within ocher deposits: The darker outer layers contain more organic material and appear as a yellowish brown dirt, producing the brawnier ochers; the yellow center layers of a deposit retain more moisture, have a finer particle size, and have the consistency of sticky cheese — producing the yellow ochers.

Crude ocher is purified by mechanical means, without synthetic intrusion. The ocher is purified by combining it with water to form a slurry, after which the sand and grit are given time to settle. The fine clay stays suspended in the water, which is finally driven off, leaving behind pure ocher.

### SOAPMAKING NOTE

If you choose to use clays, add them just before you add scent. For the best incorporation of product, add ½–1 cup (125–250 ml) clay to 1 or 2 cups (250–500 ml) ever-so-lightly traced soap, and whisk to blend before returning the mixture to the rest of the batch. Do not wait for a good trace, or you will be forced to rush the essential oils into the soap to avoid too thick a mixture.

# CHAPTER 12
## Saturated versus Unsaturated Soap Formulas

The distinction between saturated and unsaturated fats and oils is an important one to the soapmaker. This difference affects the physical and chemical characteristics of both the saponifying soap mixture and the final bars. A soapmaker who understands saturation can better visualize how the raw materials affect the finished product. In this chapter I will describe the chemistry; compare more saturated soap formulas (those that contain a high percentage of saturated fats and oils) to unsaturated formulas (those that contain a high percentage of unsaturated oils); and explain how saturation affects tracing times and the texture of the final bars. Saturation begins with saturated fatty acids and involves molecular bonding, so that is where I'll begin as well.

## SATURATION AND ATOMS AND ELECTRONS

At room temperature, most unsaturated oils are liquid and most saturated fats are solid. This is all we need to know about fats and oils to get through most of life. But once we begin to use these fats and oils to make soap, these generalizations are no longer satisfactory. We now must study atoms and their electrons to better understand saturation, for saturation is directly related to the attraction of atoms for one another.

Atoms become stable as they fill their outer shells with electrons. If a particular atom's outer shell can accommodate eight electrons but only has six, that atom seeks two more electrons, to create a full house. If an atom's outer shell can accommodate eight electrons and has two, that atom is anxious to pass along its two electrons to another atom in need of more electrons, emptying its outer shell and leaving its next inner shell full. How saturated or unsaturated a fat or an oil is relates to how its atoms have positioned themselves with other atoms in an effort to come closest to the more stable arrangements.

## Saturated Fatty Acid

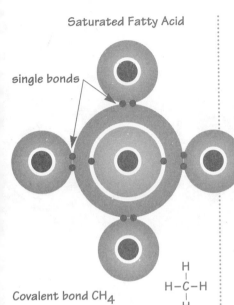

single bonds

Covalent bond $CH_4$

H
|
H–C–H
|
H

Carbon has 6 electrons
(2 in first shell, 4 in outer shell).
Hydrogen has 1 electron in the first
shell (which is also its outer shell).

## Unsaturated Fatty Acid

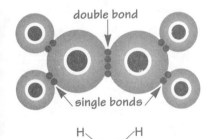

double bond

single bonds

$C_2H_4$

H       H
  \   /
   C=C
  /   \
H       H

All 4 electrons in a double bond
belong to both carbon atoms.

Those electrons available in the outer shell of an atom to be lost, gained, or shared are called valence electrons. Carbon and hydrogen atoms, the principal components of fatty acids, reach capacity by sharing electrons with one another. Carbon, which can accommodate eight valence electrons in its outer shell but has four, seeks four more electrons. Hydrogen, with one valence electron in its outer shell (it can accommodate two), needs another. A symbiotic relationship links carbon and hydrogen to one another, through the sharing of their valence electrons. This sharing is referred to as covalent bonding.

Atoms often link through ionic or covalent bonding. Think of a bond as the pull or force that holds atoms to one another. In ionic bonding, electrons are transferred from one atom to another; the attraction of opposite electrical charges holds these ionic bonds together. In covalent bonding, atoms share one or more sets of electrons, instead of transferring them. The atoms within fatty acids are held to one another through covalent bonding, as are the atoms in most organic compounds.

The sharing of one set of electrons (one electron from each atom) is known as a single bond. The sharing of two sets of electrons (two from each atom) is a double bond. Triple bonds involve the sharing of three sets of electrons. Unsaturated oils contain one or more double or triple covalent bonds. Each carbon atom within a saturated fat forms four single covalent bonds with four other atoms. Oleic acid has one double bond and is a monounsaturated (meaning one double bond) fatty acid. Linoleic, linolenic, and arachidonic acids are polyunsaturated (meaning many double bonds) fatty acids having two, three, and four double bonds. In a saturated fat, all bonds between carbon atoms are single bonds, with hydrogen atoms attached to all of the carbon atoms (except for the carbon atom in the carboxyl group, which has a double bond with one oxygen atom; see chapter 13, page 233).

At a glance, the structural formulas of saturated fats and unsaturated oils look nearly identical — long chains of carbon and hydrogen atoms with carboxyl groups at one end. An untrained eye may only notice a few more or less carbon and hydrogen atoms, and the occasional double dash instead of a single dash. Though seemingly insignificant, these single and double lines represent single and double bonds, and bonding is what determines the degree of saturation — and, ultimately, some physical characteristics of the resulting soaps.

## Saturation and Stability

Saturated fats, which are usually solid at room temperature, tend to be more stable and therefore less likely to react than unsaturated oils, because single covalent bonds are typically more stable than double or triple bonds. Unsaturated oils are more reactive than saturated compounds, since double or triple bonds are vulnerable to stray atoms seeking whatever linkages are available. These unsaturated oils are usually liquid at room temperature because their unsaturated fatty-acid chains bend at their double and triple bonds, unlike straight-chained saturated fatty acids. The atoms within linear, saturated chains are packed tightly together, but the bends, or kinks, within unsaturated chains loosen the arrangement of atoms and cause oils to be liquid at room temperature. The bends in these unsaturated chains inhibit the ability of lye to locate fatty-acid molecules quickly and easily. That is why unsaturated oils take slightly longer to saponify than saturated fats (see Chapter 13 "Breaking Down Acids," page 230 and "Molecular Weights of Fatty Acids," page 242).

Unsaturated fatty acids, being less stable, build less stable fats and oils. Again, it is the double bonds along the hydrocarbon chains that render a fatty acid unsaturated. A chain of single bonds is like a full house, packed with fully satisfied atoms. A chain containing any double bonds is likely to oxidize — a reaction in which oxygen latches onto compounds and slowly degrades their material, making it rancid. Double bonds have more room for the oxygen atoms and are more inviting than the more satisfied single bonds. Thus, unsaturated fats and oils become rancid sooner.

# HYDROGENATION

An unsaturated fatty-acid chain includes at least one pair of carbon atoms that is bonded by a double or triple bond. A chemical process called hydrogenation adds hydrogen to the double or triple bonds of fatty-acid chains, using nickel, platinum, or palladium as catalysts. In this process the multiple bonds between the carbon atoms are broken, leaving a place for a hydrogen atom to attach itself to each carbon atom. The unsaturated oil thus becomes partially or fully saturated, depending upon how many of the double bonds are affected.

Hydrogenation extends the life of fats and oils. It also affects their physical traits, such as liquidity, melting point, hardness, and tracing time. Unsaturated fatty-acid chains bend or kink slightly at their double bonds, creating looser structures; they become more liquid with more double bonds, and more solid as hydrogenation breaks those double bonds. The degree of saturation also determines melting point: Unsaturated, or partially saturated, fats and oils have lower melting points than those that are fully saturated. Double bonds in the unsaturated fatty acids render the chains, and therefore the oils and the resulting soaps, lighter, quicker to melt, and more soluble. The straighter saturated chains are more tightly packed into a solid material, adding hardness to its fats and oils and to the final bars of soap. Hydrogenated fats and oils saponify more quickly than the original, less saturated fats and oils. For instance, liquid soybean oil and liquid cottonseed oil take longer to saponify than their hydrogenated version, shortening. As the hydrogenation process converts some of the unsaturated fatty acids into saturated fatty acids, lye is better able reach and react with its mates to make soap.

## The Nature of Essential Fatty Acids

Before replacing too high a percentage of your total soapmaking fats and oils with hydrogenated fats and oils, consider a few facts about essential fatty acids.

Unsaturated vegetable oils contain unique skin-care nutrients known as essential fatty acids, once called vitamin F. These essential fatty acids include linoleic, linolenic, and arachidonic acids, all of which must be supplied to the body from outside sources, since our bodies do not manufacture them. A diet lacking in essential fatty acids causes a variety of internal damage and deficiencies, along with dry, scaling hair, skin, or scalp. These essential fatty acids are also effective topically as a moisturizer when applied to dry skin and hair. Though all fatty acids are emollient, the essential fatty acids are thought to be especially so.

Unfortunately, the hydrogenation process, which occurs at temperatures of between 200°F and 275°F (93°C and 135°C), oxidizes and destroys the essential fatty acids as well as the fat-soluble vitamins found in the unsaturated oils. So, while hydrogenation postpones spoilage and creates harder fats and oils, it also degrades the fats and oils and robs them of some unique skin-care properties. The hydrogenated fats and oils will still give the soap lather, texture, and hardness — and even moisturizing qualities — but their fullest offering is forfeited.

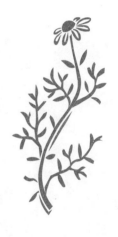

## BALANCING THE PERCENTAGES OF SATURATED AND UNSATURATED FATS AND OILS

My favorite cold-process soap incorporates a carefully calculated combination of saturated fats and unsaturated oils. Degree of saturation affects a soap's hardness, lather, trace time, texture, and feel in water. A formula that combines the finest attributes of each fat or oil, saturated and unsaturated, creates a soap with an optimum blend of traits. Since I prefer the skin-care properties of soaps made with at least 30 percent unsaturated oils, I limit the use of hydrogenated or naturally saturated fats and oils. In my basic soap, olive oil (which is unsaturated) constitutes around 40 percent of my total fats and oils; the balance is palm oil (which is naturally saturated) and coconut oil (which is naturally saturated and/or hydrogenated).

## Saturated Fats and Oils and Their Soaps

Some soapmakers prefer formulas that incorporate high percentages of hydrogenated and/or naturally saturated fats and oils for the quickest trace and the hardest soap. Often these supersaturated batches are produced at higher temperatures, to accommodate the higher melting points and solidification points of saturated fats and oils. Such high soapmaking temperatures mean only a short wait before the cooling oils and fats and the lye solution reach the desired temperatures. Saturated formulas can be produced at a temperature range of 90–140°F (32–60°C); I like the 90–100°F range (32–38°C). Keep in mind that some formulas made at over 130°F (54.4°C) require slightly more water to allow for evaporation, and must be stirred very quickly to avoid curdling.

For the benefit of soapmakers looking for more saturated blends, I've included many formulas in chapter 1 that blend a high percentage of saturated fats and oils with what I consider to be a desirable percentage of unsaturated oils.

# CHAPTER 13
## The Chemistry of Soapmaking

In *The Natural Soap Book*, I offered an introduction to the chemistry of soapmaking. In an effort not to overwhelm the beginner, I discussed the most relevant chemical terms as generally as possible. My goal was to give a method to reach desired results without necessarily understanding all of the underlying chemistry. This chapter is for those who want to be overwhelmed.

There are many different ways to produce soap, using a variety of raw materials. Since the technical definition of *soap* includes even those products with no soaplike properties, some "soaps" look and feel little or nothing like our favorite bar soaps. But all soaps have something in common — they are all produced when a fatty acid and a base react. This product of the reaction is a slightly acidic salt called soap.

The box on the next page presents seven equations. Each represents soapmaking, but only equation #7 represents the cold-process method used to make soap at home. It is this process that I will discuss in detail in this chapter. The other six formulas relate to industrial soapmaking.

## What Is Soap?

*Soap* is defined as the product that results from the reaction of a fatty acid and a strong base. Some soaps that satisfy this definition have nothing to do with cleansing. Most bath soaps are made using the alkali sodium hydroxide, but soap can also be made using a variety of bases, to create a variety of unrecognizable products. Some are made with organic alkalis, such as ammonia or amines (ammonia derivatives, such as triethanolamine). Soap-emulsified petrochemicals are used to make synthetic rubber. Metallic soaps are made with nonalkali metals such as copper, calcium, and zinc, and are used to inhibit metallic corrosion, to waterproof textiles, and to mildew-proof leather. Chemically, these are

## SEVEN REACTIONS THAT PRODUCE SOAP

**#1: Pure fatty acid reacts with sodium hydroxide to form sodium soap**

$$2CH_3 - (CH_2)_{16} - COOH + \quad NaOH \quad \rightarrow CH_3(CH_2)_{16} - COONa + H_2O$$

    stearic acid     + sodium hydroxide →    sodium soap    + water

**#2: Pure fatty acid reacts with a carbonate to form sodium soap**

$$2CH_3 - (CH_2)_{16} - COOH + \quad Na_2CO_3 \quad \rightarrow 2CH_3 - (CH_2)_{16} - COONa + CO_2 + H_2O$$

    stearic acid     + sodium carbonate →    sodium soap    + carbon + water
                                                            dioxide

**#3: Triglyceride reacts with potassium hydroxide to form liquid potassium soap**

$$C_3H_5(C_{18}H_{35}O_2)_3 + \quad 3KOH \quad \rightarrow C_3H_5(OH)_3 + 3KC_{18}H_{35}O_2$$

    tristearin     + potassium hydroxide →    glycerin    + potassium stearate

**#4: Triglyceride reacts with sodium hydroxide to form sodium soap**

$$C_3H_5(C_{18}H_{35}5O_2)_3 + \quad 3NaOH \quad \rightarrow 3NaC_{18}H_{35}O_2 + C_3H_5(OH)_3$$

    stearin     + sodium hydroxide → sodium stearate +    glycerin

**#5: Fatty acid reacts with ammonia to form amide soap**

$$RCOOH + \quad NH_3 \quad \rightarrow RCONH_2 + H_2O$$

fatty acid + ammonia →    amide    + water

**#6: Fatty acid reacts with an amine (an ammonia derivative) to form amide soap**

$$RNH_2 + R'COOH \quad \rightarrow RCONHR' + H_2O$$

amine + fatty acid →    amide    + water

**#7: Triglyceride reacts with sodium hydroxide to form sodium soap**

  COOR                             OH

$$C_3H_5COOR + \quad 3NaOH \quad \rightarrow C_3H_5OH + 3NaCOOR$$

  COOR                             OH

triglyceride + sodium hydroxide → glycerin + sodium soap

**Note:** R, R', and R" stands for primary, secondary, and tertiary. These are all fancy names for different fatty-acid chains with varying numbers of carbon and hydrogen atoms.

all soaps. Still, I speak of a very different kind of soap in this book: cold-process soap, which means that once the heated fats and oils are mixed with the lye solution, only the heat of the reaction (without the addition of any external heat) drives the soapmaking process forward.

## What Is Saponification?

Saponification is another name for soapmaking. The simplest saponification process is cold-process soapmaking, defined above. Chemically, when an acid and a base combine, they form a salt. In cold-process soapmaking, the slightly acidic fats and oils react with the highly basic sodium hydroxide to create gentle soap, a slightly basic salt. In fact, the typical dictionary definition of soap is "the salt of a fatty acid and a metal."

Some acids do not burn, including the fats and oils used to make soap, and some salts, including the soaps we bathe with, have nothing to do with sodium chloride, the spice of life. *Salt* refers not only to the deposits left in the oceans and seas, commonly known as sodium chloride, but also to the compound formed when a metal replaces the hydrogen in an acid. The metal — the sodium in sodium hydroxide — replaces hydrogen in the fatty-acid portion of the fat or oil to create soap, known chemically as a salt.

## THE SAPONIFICATION PROCESS

The chemistry of soapmaking should be perceived as two separate processes: (A) the breaking down of ingredients into useful parts; and (B) the reaction of the useful parts to form soap. This chapter explains both processes in detail.

The first process — the breaking down of ingredients — actually refers to two subprocesses: (1) the breaking down of fats and oils into fatty acids; and (2) the splitting apart of sodium hydroxide to generate hydroxide ions and sodium ions.

Fats and oils consist of triglycerides. You cannot make soap out of triglycerides. Rather, you have to break down the triglycerides into their useful parts: fatty acids and glycerol. Fatty acids are absolutely critical to the soapmaking process. Glycerol is not a vital component, but it is helpful and worthwhile. The process of breaking down triglycerides into fatty acids and glycerol is called hydrolysis, and is discussed in detail in the following section.

Sodium hydroxide also needs to be broken down. What is essential to soapmaking is the hydroxide ion. The breaking down of sodium hydroxide into hydroxide ions and sodium ions is called ionization.

Water is important to both of the subprocesses. Water, as part of an alkaline solution, will break down a triglyceride. It will also permit ionization of sodium hydroxide.

The second process — the reaction of the useful parts — actually refers to two reactions: (1) the reaction of fatty acids and sodium ions to produce soap; and (2) the reaction of glycerol and the hydroxide ion to form glycerin. Water is important to both reactions even though it does not itself chemically react: It is the medium in which the useful parts can flow, mix, and react.

The two processes together — the breaking down of ingredients into useful parts and the reaction of useful parts to form soap — constitute saponification.

## The Breaking-Down Processes

This refers to the breaking down both of the acids (fats and oils into fatty acids) and of the bases (sodium hydroxide into sodium and hydroxide).

**Breaking Down Acids.** Fats and oils consist of triglycerides. Triglycerides consist of fatty acids and glycerol. Fatty acids are long hydrocarbon chains attached to carboxyl groups. The process of breaking down triglycerides into fatty acids is called hydrolysis. Let's examine each of these statements in more detail.

*Fats and oils consist of triglycerides.* Each fat and oil consists of a different combination of triglycerides — compounds made up of three fatty acids linked to one molecule of glycerol. In addition, fats and oils also include so-called free fatty acids (fatty acids not linked to glycerol). When you melt solid fats and oils, the result is a pool of triglycerides and some free fatty acids.

*Triglycerides consist of fatty acids and glycerol.* For example, olein is a triglyceride consisting of three molecules of oleic acid (one kind of fatty acid) and one molecule of glycerol. There are more than seventy different fatty acids, and nearly all of them are straight chains of carbon and hydrogen atoms with even numbers of carbon atoms. Each fat and oil consists of different combinations of various fatty acids, with the predominant fatty acids determining that oil's soapmaking characteristics. The charts beginning on page 238 indicate which soap characteristics are contributed by each fatty acid and which fatty acids are in each oil.

Fatty acids can be saturated or unsaturated (see chapter 12, "Saturated versus Unsaturated Soap Formulas"). In a saturated fatty acid, the carbon atoms are bonded with single bonds. They share one set of electrons. Fats that contain a high percentage of saturated fatty acids are usually solid at room temperature. Unsaturated fatty acids contain at least one double bond — one set of carbon atoms bonded by the sharing of two sets of electrons. Fats and oils that contain a high percentage of unsaturated fatty acids are usually liquid at room temperature. Triglycerides contain two or three different fatty acids; fats and oils are as saturated or unsaturated as the combined saturated nature of their constituent fatty acids.

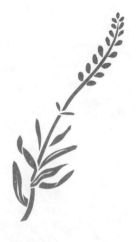

The physical characteristics of fats and oils are determined by the arrangement of the fatty acids in the triglycerides. The structures are definite arrangements of hydrogen and carbon atoms, with numbers assigned to each carbon atom along the chain. Saturated fats have saturated fatty acids positioned on particular carbon atoms. Unsaturated fats and oils have unsaturated fatty acids in those positions. For instance, lard has palmitic acid — a saturated fatty acid — positioned on the second or middle carbon atom of the glyceride. Vegetable oils have unsaturated fatty acids in this position, with saturated fatty acids on the end carbons of the glyceride. The geometric configurations of the saturated and unsaturated fatty acids are sometimes labeled trans- or cis-. A cis- double bond, one kind of arrangement, produces bends in the molecules, resulting in less molecular attraction between atoms and a less-solid, unsaturated material. A transconfiguration, a different geometic arrangement, produces a more packed, linear structure with greater intermolecular force. This tighter arrangement is more solid and saturated (see page 242, "Molecular Weights of Fatty Acids").

## PALMITIC ACID (Saturated Fatty Acid)
## $C_{16}H_{32}O_2$

$$H-\overset{\overset{\displaystyle H}{|}}{\underset{\underset{\displaystyle H}{|}}{C}}-\overset{\overset{\displaystyle H}{|}}{\underset{\underset{\displaystyle H}{|}}{C}}-\overset{\overset{\displaystyle H}{|}}{\underset{\underset{\displaystyle H}{|}}{C}}-\overset{\overset{\displaystyle H}{|}}{\underset{\underset{\displaystyle H}{|}}{C}}-\overset{\overset{\displaystyle H}{|}}{\underset{\underset{\displaystyle H}{|}}{C}}-\overset{\overset{\displaystyle H}{|}}{\underset{\underset{\displaystyle H}{|}}{C}}-\overset{\overset{\displaystyle H}{|}}{\underset{\underset{\displaystyle H}{|}}{C}}-\overset{\overset{\displaystyle H}{|}}{\underset{\underset{\displaystyle H}{|}}{C}}-\overset{\overset{\displaystyle H}{|}}{\underset{\underset{\displaystyle H}{|}}{C}}-\overset{\overset{\displaystyle H}{|}}{\underset{\underset{\displaystyle H}{|}}{C}}-\overset{\overset{\displaystyle H}{|}}{\underset{\underset{\displaystyle H}{|}}{C}}-\overset{\overset{\displaystyle H}{|}}{\underset{\underset{\displaystyle H}{|}}{C}}-\overset{\overset{\displaystyle H}{|}}{\underset{\underset{\displaystyle H}{|}}{C}}-\overset{\overset{\displaystyle H}{|}}{\underset{\underset{\displaystyle H}{|}}{C}}-\overset{\overset{\displaystyle H}{|}}{\underset{\underset{\displaystyle H}{|}}{C}}-\overset{\overset{\displaystyle O}{\parallel}}{C}-OH$$

Hydrogen end is not soluble in water.  Carboxyl end is soluble in water.

*Fatty acids consist of hydrocarbon chains with a carboxyl group at the end.* Fatty acids are long chains of carbon, hydrogen, and oxygen atoms. For example, oleic acid is a fatty acid consisting of eighteen carbon atoms, thirty-four hydrogen atoms, and two oxygen atoms. Carbon easily forms covalent bonds with other carbon atoms in long chains and rings, explaining how such long fatty-acid chains as the oleic-acid are possible.

## OLEIC ACID (Unsaturated Fatty Acid)
## $C_{18}H_{34}O_2$

$$H-\overset{\overset{\displaystyle H}{|}}{\underset{\underset{\displaystyle H}{|}}{C}}-\overset{\overset{\displaystyle H}{|}}{\underset{\underset{\displaystyle H}{|}}{C}}-\overset{\overset{\displaystyle H}{|}}{\underset{\underset{\displaystyle H}{|}}{C}}-\overset{\overset{\displaystyle H}{|}}{\underset{\underset{\displaystyle H}{|}}{C}}-\overset{\overset{\displaystyle H}{|}}{\underset{\underset{\displaystyle H}{|}}{C}}-\overset{\overset{\displaystyle H}{|}}{\underset{\underset{\displaystyle H}{|}}{C}}-\overset{\overset{\displaystyle H}{|}}{\underset{\underset{\displaystyle H}{|}}{C}}-\overset{\overset{\displaystyle H}{|}}{C}=\overset{\overset{\displaystyle H}{|}}{C}-\overset{\overset{\displaystyle H}{|}}{\underset{\underset{\displaystyle H}{|}}{C}}-\overset{\overset{\displaystyle H}{|}}{\underset{\underset{\displaystyle H}{|}}{C}}-\overset{\overset{\displaystyle H}{|}}{\underset{\underset{\displaystyle H}{|}}{C}}-\overset{\overset{\displaystyle H}{|}}{\underset{\underset{\displaystyle H}{|}}{C}}-\overset{\overset{\displaystyle H}{|}}{\underset{\underset{\displaystyle H}{|}}{C}}-\overset{\overset{\displaystyle H}{|}}{\underset{\underset{\displaystyle H}{|}}{C}}-\overset{\overset{\displaystyle O}{\parallel}}{C}-OH$$

carboxyl group

A fatty acid is formed when a chain of hydrogen and carbon atoms (no oxygen), known as an alkane, drops one of its hydrogen atoms (at which point it is known as an alkyl group), and replaces the missing hydrogen atom with a group consisting of one carbon atom, two oxygen atoms, and one hydrogen atom (known as a carboxyl group, represented symbolically as COOH). In other words, when an alkyl group joins with a carboxyl group, the result is a fatty acid, also known as a carboxylic acid. In the above-depicted structural formula for oleic acid, the carboxyl group (COOH) is attached to the alkyl group at the right end.

Remember that when three fatty acids combine with glycerol (represented symbolically as $C_3H_5$), the result is a triglyceride.

*A triglyceride is one kind of ester; all esters can be saponified.* Esters are compounds formed when acids react with alcohols in the presence of water. Triglycerides are esters — composed of fatty acids (the acid) and glycerol (the alcohol) — which is why they saponify to form soap. But the category of esters includes more than triglycerides. It also includes such other substances as beeswax, lanolin, and lecithin, to name a few. These other esters contain different kinds of acids and alcohols from the ones in triglycerides, but they too saponify.

In the reaction that forms a triglyceride — a neutral fat — each of the three OH groups in the glycerin reacts with each of the three fatty acids. For the carboxylic acid to become an ester, the OH from the carboxyl group (see diagram at right) of each fatty acid is released, three H atoms from the alcohol are released, and the OHs and Hs combine to form water. The remaining atoms in the carboxylic acid join to form the ester, a carboxylic acid minus the OH in the carboxyl group. When the carboxylic acid reacts with alcohol, an alkyl group is left attached to the double-bonded oxygen from the old carboxyl group, producing a triglyceride (the fatty acids combined with glycerol), plus water (see diagram at right).

*Hydrolysis is the process that breaks down fats and oils into useful parts.* All esters, including glycerides, can be split by the absorption of water into their components, glycerin and an acid. The splitting of triglyceride into its constituent bodies is called hydrolysis. In the following formula, tristearin is a triglyceride and stearic acid is a fatty acid.

$$C_3H_5(C_{18}H_{35}O_2)_3 + 3H_2O = C_3H_5(OH)_3 + 3HC_{18}H_{35}O_2$$

| tristearin | water | glycerin | stearic acid |

$$
\begin{array}{c}
O \\
\parallel \\
C\!-\!O\,H
\end{array}
$$

The structural formula of the carboxyl group.

$$
\begin{array}{c}
O \\
\parallel \\
C\!-\! \text{alkyl group}
\end{array}
$$
(hydrocarbon chain)

The structural formula of the carboxyl group within the triglyceride, missing the OH.

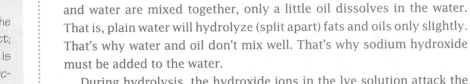
The water in a soapmaking formula carries the sodium hydroxide to all corners of the pan, and then participates in hydrolysis. When fats and water are mixed together, only a little oil dissolves in the water. That is, plain water will hydrolyze (split apart) fats and oils only slightly. That's why water and oil don't mix well. That's why sodium hydroxide must be added to the water.

During hydrolysis, the hydroxide ions in the lye solution attack the carbon in the carboxyl end of the fatty acids, breaking off one fatty acid at a time from the triglyceride. Each released fatty acid is then free to react with the sodium ion to make soap. Three hydroxide ions react with the glycerol to make glycerin.

Hydrolysis proceeds in three different stages. First, the water and sodium hydroxide solution act upon the triglyceride and split it into a diglyceride — two fatty acids and glycerol — freeing one fatty acid which is then available to react with sodium to make soap. This little bit of soap made during the first stage acts as an emulsifier and pulls other components into the soapmaking reaction. During the second stage, the

### During Hydrolysis:

1. The OH ion (from the sodium hydroxide) attacks the carbon in the carboxyl portion of each fatty acid, breaking off one fatty acid at a time from the triglyceride, then the diglyceride, then finally, the monoglyceride.
2. Each released fatty acid reacts with the sodium ion to make soap.
3. The OH ions react with glycerol ($C_3H_5$) to make glycerin ($C_3H_5OH_3$).

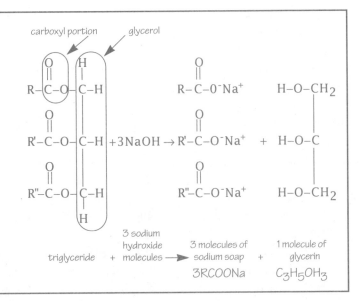

water and sodium hydroxide solution split the diglyceride into a mono-glyceride — one fatty acid and glycerol — freeing up another fatty acid to make more soap. Finally, in the third stage, the water and sodium hydroxide solution split the monoglyceride into glycerol and a separate fatty acid, completing the conversion of the original triglyceride into its separate fatty acids and free glycerol. The free glycerol reacts with three hydroxide molecules from the lye solution to form glycerin.

*The Hydrolysis of unsaturates is slower.* The atoms within an unsaturated triglyceride are less orderly than those within a saturated triglyceride. Unsaturated oils have more double bonds. Since hydrocarbon chains bend at their double bonds, twisting and sending portions of the chains off at angles from the straight chain, unsaturated oils have more irregular shapes. If you imagine single-bonded saturates as two-dimensional sheets of paper stacked in a pile, then imagine double-bonded unsaturates as three-dimensional crumpled paper, which you could carry only in a gunnysack. This arrangement creates a less compact unit, since the atoms are not all held tightly together. Unsaturated triglycerides are normally liquid at room temperature. When these chains bend and twist around themselves into more contorted configurations, it becomes harder for the sodium hydroxide to position itself for a reaction. Therefore, unsaturated oils take longer to saponify than do saturated fats and oils. See chapter 12 for a more detailed discussion of saturated versus unsaturated soap formulas.

**Breaking Down Bases:** Fats and oils cannot be converted into soap without the presence of a base. A variety of bases can be used to make soap, but in cold-process soapmaking the most common is sodium hydroxide. Some of the formulas listed at the beginning of this chapter incorporate other bases, such as potassium hydroxide, sodium carbonate, ammonia, and amines. Some of these are alkalis, compounds of a metal ion and a hydroxide ion ($OH^-$); some are not alkalis.

An alkali is a hydroxide of one of the alkali metals, those elements on the far left side of the periodic chart with just one electron in their outer shells — lithium, sodium, potassium, rubidium, caesium. The addition of a hydroxide group (OH⁻) to the alkali metals creates hydroxides of the metals. For example, sodium hydroxide, NaOH, is the hydroxide of the metal sodium. Lithium hydroxide is the hydroxide of the metal lithium. All alkalis in solution (dissolved in water) increase the hydroxide ion concentration.

Sodium hydroxide is the base used to make a cold-process soap, and other types as well. Sodium alone would not combine with water to make lye; sodium hydroxide, NaOH, is what combines with water to make the lye solution.

Sodium hydroxide is a combination of one sodium ion and one hydroxide ion. The hydroxide ion consists of one oxygen atom and one hydrogen atom. It is the hydroxide ion, not the sodium ion, that is most critical to soapmaking. Other bases could be used in place of sodium hydroxide, because, again, it is the hydroxide ion that drives the process of hydrolysis.

When sodium hydroxide is added to water, the sodium ions are split apart from the hydroxide ions. This process is called ionization and releases heat. The result is free $Na^+$ ions and $OH^-$ ions, which are then available to react.

## The Reaction Processes

This refers to the reaction both of the fatty acids and sodium to form soap, and of the glycerol and hydroxide to form glycerin.

**The Reaction of Fatty Acids and Sodium to Produce Soap:** As triglycerides break down into fatty acids and glycerols, the fatty acids become available to react with the sodium ions in the lye solution. The result is soap.

I have rather artificially divided soapmaking into the breaking-down processes and the reaction processes. I think this is helpful conceptually, but it is somewhat misleading. Contrary to the image, the two processes occur simultaneously, each contributing to the other.

**The Reaction of Glycerol and the Hydroxide Ion to Produce Glycerin:** As triglycerides break down into fatty acids and glycerols, the glycerol becomes available to react with the hydroxide ions in the lye solution. The result is glycerin.

$$C_3H_5 + 3OH \rightarrow C_3H_5(OH)_3$$
glycerol    hydroxide    glycerin

Glycerin is a marvelous additive that moisturizes the skin. Industrial manufacturers either remove this glycerin and sell it as a by-product, or make soap with free fatty acids (without glycerol attached) rather than with triglycerides (which include glycerol).

## USING CHEMISTRY TO MAKE BETTER SOAP

As I warned you in the introduction to this book, I like to understand as much as possible, even if the knowledge may not prove to be useful. However, this does not mean that the foregoing academic discussion of the chemistry of soapmaking is not useful in the kitchen. To the contrary, chemistry can improve your soapmaking: It allows you to manipulate soap characteristics by choosing fats and oils with certain fatty acids, and by examining molecular weights; it allows you to calculate how much sodium hydroxide you'll need to saponify a given amount of fats and oils; and it allows you to anticipate and perhaps avoid rancidity.

### Examining the Constituent Fatty Acids

The major characteristics we look for in a soap — the hardness of the bar, the fluffiness of the lather, and the stability of the lather — depend upon which fatty acids are used to make it. Each fat or oil is a unique combination of several different fatty acids. The characteristics contributed by a particular fat or oil are determined by the characteristics of its predominant fatty acid(s). For example, palm oil consists of 40.1 percent palmitic acid — a fatty acid that increases the hardness of a bar. That's

**DEFINING LYE**

*Lye* has two meanings: It is the solid form of a caustic alkali; and it is also the water solution in which a caustic alkali has been dissolved. Technically, *lye* has a narrower meaning than *alkali* or *base*, and a broader meaning than *caustic soda*. I most often call sodium hydroxide "sodium hydroxide," and the sodium hydroxide/water solution "lye." The lye solution is a slippery, strongly alkaline substance. It is this base that reacts with fats and oils to make soap.

why palm oil is known for contributing to a hard soap. Once you know the fatty-acid makeup of the fats or oils in a soap formula, you can figure out what characteristics the soap will have. You need two charts for this, as follow. The first chart identifies which soap characteristics are contributed by the more common fatty acids. The second indicates which fatty acids are in each fat and oil.

As the charts indicate, no one fat or oil has all of the characteristics soapmakers find desirable. Thus, we must combine different fats and oils to produce the outcome we desire. This is where our skill and artistry as soapmakers are most tested.

## SOAP CHARACTERISTICS PRODUCED BY VARIOUS FATTY ACIDS

| Fatty Acid | Hard Bar | Cleansing | Fluffy Lather | Conditioning | Stable Lather |
|---|---|---|---|---|---|
| Lauric | X | X | X | | |
| Linoleic | | | | X | |
| Myristic | X | X | X | | |
| Oleic | | | | X | |
| Palmitic | X | | | | X |
| Ricinoleic | | | X | X | X |
| Stearic | X | | | | X |

## THE FATTY ACID MAKEUP OF SOME COMMON FATS AND OILS

| Fat or Oil | Fatty Acids (in percentages) |
| --- | --- |
| Almond (Sweet) Oil | Oleic (69.4), linoleic (17.4), stearic (6.5) arachidic (1.7), palmitoleic (0.6), other (4.4) |
| Avocado Oil | Oleic (62.0), linoleic (16.0), myristic (15.2), palmitic (5.5), linolenic (1.0), stearic (0.13) |
| Babassu Oil | Lauric (44.1), oleic (16.1) myristic (15.4), palmitic (8.5), capric (6.6), caprylic (4.8), stearic (2.7), linoleic (1.4), arachidic (0.2), caproic (0.2) |
| Beef Tallow | Oleic (42.0), palmitic (29.0), stearic (20.0), myristic (3.0), linoleic (2.0), other (4.0) |
| Borage Oil | Linoleic (38.1), linolenic (25.1), oleic (14.2), palmitic (9.4), stearic (2.8), arachidic (0.7), palmitoleic (0.5), other (9.2) |
| Canola/Rapeseed Oil | Erucic (50.0), oleic (32.0), linoleic (15.0), palmitic (1.0), linolenic (1.0), other (1.0) |
| Castor Oil | Ricinoleic (87.0), oleic (7.0), linoleic (3.0), palmitic (2.0), stearic (1.0) |
| Cocoa Butter | Oleic (38.1), stearic (35.4), palmitic (24.4), linoleic (2.1) |
| Coconut Oil | Lauric (48.0), myristic (17.0), palmitic (9.0), caprylic (8.0), capric (7.0), oleic (6.0), stearic (2.0), linoleic (2.0), caproic (0.5), palmitoleic (0.2), other (0.3) |
| Corn Oil | Oleic (49.6), linoleic (34.3), palmitic (10.2), stearic (3.0), palmitoleic (1.5), myristic (1.4) |
| Evening Primrose Oil | Linoleic (70.6), oleic (11.2), linolenic (9.4), palmitic (6.1), stearic (1.6), palmitoleic (0.2), other (0.9) |
| Hazelnut Oil | Oleic (77.8), linoleic (14.5), palmitic (5.2), stearic (2.0), palmitoleic (0.2), myristic (0.1), other (0.2) |

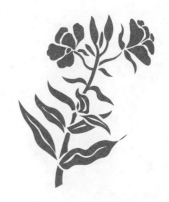

### A NOTE ON THIS CHART
Fatty acid breakdowns can vary from lot to lot, and some unidentified trace elements can add up to a few percentage points, so no chart of this type is exact.

*continued on next page*

## THE FATTY ACID MAKEUP OF SOME COMMON FATS AND OILS (cont'd.)

| Fat or Oil | Fatty Acids (in percentages) |
|---|---|
| Kukui Nut Oil | Linoleic (43.6), linolenic (33.2), oleic (13.9), palmitic (6.4), stearic (0.3), other (2.6) |
| Lard | Oleic (46.0), palmitic (28.0), stearic (13.0), linoleic (6.0), palmitoleic (3.0), myristic (1.0), myristoleic (0.2), other (2.8) |
| Macadamia Nut Oil | Oleic (57.8), palmitoleic (21.4), palmitic (8.8), linolenic (3.4), linoleic (2.7), arachidic (2.6), stearic (2.5), myristic (0.8) |
| Mutton Tallow | Oleic (36.0), stearic (30.5), palmitic (24.6), myristic (4.6), linoleic (4.3) |
| Olive Oil | Oleic (84.4), palmitic (6.9), stearic (2.3), linoleic (4.6), arachidic (0.1), myristic (trace), other (1.7) |
| Palm Kernel Oil | Lauric (46.9), oleic (18.5), myristic (14.1), palmitic (8.8), capric (7.0), caprylic (2.7), stearic (1.3), linoleic (0.7) |
| Palm Oil | Oleic (42.7), palmitic (40.1), linoleic (10.3), stearic (5.5), myristic (1.4) |
| Peanut Oil | Oleic (56.0), linoleic (26.0), palmitic (8.3), stearic (3.1), behenic (3.1), arachidic (2.4), lignoceric (1.1) |
| Safflower Oil | Linoleic (70.1), oleic (18.6), linolenic (3.4), combined total of lauric, myristic, palmitic, stearic, and arachidic (7.9) |
| Sesame Oil | Linoleic (41.3), oleic (39.3), palmitic (8.9), stearic (4.8), linolenic (0.3), palmitoleic (0.2), other (5.2) |
| Soybean Oil | Linoleic (50.7), oleic (28.9), palmitic (9.8), linolenic (6.5), stearic (2.4), arachidic (0.9), palmitoleic (0.4), lauric (0.2), myristic (0.1), C14 monoethenoic (0.1) |
| Sunflower Seed Oil | Linoleic (66.2), oleic (25.1), palmitic (5.6), stearic (2.2), arachidic (0.9) |
| Wheat Germ Oil | Linoleic (52.3), oleic (28.1), linolenic (3.6), combined total of lauric, myristic, palmitic, stearic, and arachidic (16.0) |

## Examining the Molecular Weights of the Constituent Fatty Acids

If you know the molecular weight of a fatty acid in your soap, often you can predict that soap's lathering ability. In general, the greater the molecular weight of a fatty acid, the less fluffy and the more stable the lather. For example, beef tallow makes a thin lather. It consists of 24.6 percent palmitic acid and 30.5 percent stearic acid, both of which have relatively high molecular weights — 256 and 284, respectively.

The molecular-weight chart on page 242 can help predict other soap characteristics as well. In general, the following observations can be trusted:

♦ Medium-molecular-weight fatty acids (capric and lauric fatty acids, which are present in coconut, palm kernel, and babassu oil) can be somewhat irritating to the skin. A limited percentage of these oils contributes a light, quick lather and is moisturizing, but in excess, they are drying. Aim for a carefully calculated blend.

♦ With increasing molecular weight, the solubility of soap decreases and the soap bar lasts longer.

♦ As the molecular weight of fatty acids increases, their lathering ability decreases. Coconut oil soaps lather well in seawater because the high proportion of lauric acid (a lower-molecular-weight fatty acid) produces a lather even in the presence of salt water. Tallow soap (tallow contains higher-weight fatty acids) does not lather well in salt water.

♦ With increasing molecular weight, the bubbles within the lather become smaller. Though the lower-molecular-weight fatty acids produce quick, fluffy lathers, these lathers are less stable. The high-molecular-weight fatty acids produce thin lathers, but the lathers last longer.

♦ With increasing molecular weight, cleansing capability decreases, along with skin irritation.

♦ The higher the molecular weight, the harder the soap, with the exception of coconut, palm kernel, and babassu oils. Though these have lower molecular weights, they still produce hard soaps by virtue of their saturated makeups.

## MOLECULAR WEIGHTS OF FATTY ACIDS

| Fatty Acid | Formula | Molecular Weight |
|---|---|---|
| Butyric | $C_4H_8O_2$ | 88 |
| Caproic | $C_6H_{12}O_2$ | 116 |
| Capric | $C_{10}H_{20}O_2$ | 172 |
| Lauric | $C_{12}H_{24}O_2$ | 200 |
| Myristic | $C_{14}H_{28}O_2$ | 228 |
| Palmitic | $C_{16}H_{32}O_2$ | 256 |
| Linoleic | $C_{18}H_{32}O_2$ | 280 |
| Oleic | $C_{18}H_{34}O_2$ | 282 |
| Stearic | $C_{18}H_{36}O_2$ | 284 |
| Ricinoleic | $C_{18}H_{34}O_3$ | 298 |
| Erucic | $C_{22}H_{42}O_2$ | 339 |

## USING SAPONIFICATION VALUE

The saponification value (referred to as the SAP value) of a particular oil is a measure of the amount of KOH (potassium hydroxide) in milligrams required to saponify 1 gram of that oil. Each fat or oil has a saponification value. The SAP value is actually a range of numbers, but the average of these numbers is usually presented on a chart. The values were determined years ago, using KOH as the base, so today's soapmaker must do some simple arithmetic to convert the measurements to NaOH. Understanding SAP value and how to derive it enables you to substitute one oil for another, and to adjust your amount of sodium hydroxide accordingly.

Oils and fats and their fatty-acid chains have different molecular weights, depending upon how many carbon, oxygen, and hydrogen atoms they have within their triglycerides. The molecular weight of a

## AN EXCEPTION TO THE RULE ON MOLECULAR WEIGHT

Coconut oil is a saturated fat with a low molecular weight — an anomaly. It is also one of the three most important soapmaking oils.

Normally, the higher the molecular weight of a saturated fatty acid, the higher its melting point and the less soluble it is in water. The more unsaturated fats and oils have lower melting points and are more soluble in water. But clearly, coconut oil soaps are very soluble and produce luscious light lathers. This is related to something highly technical and complicated.

The structural configuration of the oil molecule determines more about the oil and its soap than does saturation alone. Most saturated fat molecules are straight-chained, and most unsaturated oil molecules branch out at their double bonds. But some unsaturated fatty acids are different: They bend and twist around themselves at their double bonds, compacting their atoms into a smaller space, instead of branching out. These variations are called isomers, and further divided into cis-isomers and trans-isomers. When the hydrocarbon chains are on one side of the double bond, the structure is a cis-isomer. When they veer off in opposing directions, the structure is a trans-isomer.

fatty acid is the total weight of the combined atoms. The molecular weight of the triglyceride is the combined weight of the fatty acids and the glycerin. The higher the molecular weight of a particular oil or fat, the less alkali (sodium hydroxide) is required to saponify it.

Saponification value represents the amount of KOH for a full saponification. For a full saponification, each molecule of oil reacts with a molecule of alkali, leaving no excess fat or alkali in the final soap. I prefer to use less sodium hydroxide than the SAP value determines, leaving an excess of fats and oils in the final bars after all of the lye has reacted. The unsaponified oils serve as moisturizing ingredients. These soaps are known as superfatted. A superfatted soap formula must be carefully calculated, however, to avoid too much of an excess of oils. This oil causes premature spoilage, known as rancidity.

You can use the SAP value of an oil or fat to determine the weight of *potassium* hydroxide required for saponification: Divide the SAP value by 1,000; then multiply the result by the weight of the oil. For example, the SAP value of olive oil is 189.7. This means that 189.7 milligrams of potassium hydroxide are required to completely saponify 1 gram (1,000 milligrams) of olive oil; 948.5 milligrams are required for 5 grams of olive oil (.1897 x 5,000). The higher the SAP value, the more base is required for saponification.

**To Calculate Sodium Hydroxide:** You can also use the SAP value to determine how much *sodium* hydroxide (NaOH) is required for saponification, with some simple arithmetic and an understanding of basic soapmaking chemistry. Saponification is affected by the number of hydroxide ions in the solution. One molecule of sodium hydroxide (NaOH) has the same number of hydroxide ions (one) as one molecule of potassium hydroxide (KOH), but since KOH is heavier than NaOH, saponification requires less (by weight) NaOH. More precisely, because the molecular weight of NaOH is 40 and the molecular weight of KOH is 56.1, the required weight of NaOH is 40/56.1 of the required weight of KOH.

Weight of NaOH required = 40/56.1 x weight of KOH required

In other words, multiply the required weight of KOH by 40, and divide the result by 56.1. In the case of olive oil, for instance, 1 gram of oil would require 135.3 milligrams of NaOH (189.7 x 40 ÷ 56.1).

## Adjusting Calculations to Produce a Superfatted Soap

So far, the science and mathematics are reassuringly precise. Unfortunately, there is one additional complication that introduces some uncertainty. The above formula indicates how much sodium hydroxide is required to completely saponify an oil. However, the soapmaker does not want to completely saponify the fats and oils — you want some fat and oil to remain unsaponified. This makes the soap milder, less caustic, and more soothing.

Our skin's mantle is slightly acidic, anywhere between 4.00 and 6.75 on the pH scale (with pH 7 being neutral). Though our skin can tolerate a wide range of pH values, including some of the alkaline values, too much sodium hydroxide can be harsh. By using less sodium hydroxide than the SAP values suggest, and an excess of oils and nutrients, your bars will be left with unsaponified oil within — making them gentle and moisturizing.

The question is, how much less sodium hydroxide should be used? That is, after applying the formula and determining the precise amount of sodium hydroxide needed for complete saponification, how much should that precise amount then be discounted? I cannot give you a neat answer here. I've searched for a single discount I could apply consistently, but haven't come up with one. I've worked with discounts ranging from 7 percent to 20 percent. The bigger the discount, the less base is used, resulting in a milder soap — that will also become rancid more quickly. When I do my calculations for a new soap formula, I usually begin with a 10 percent superfatting discount. In *The Natural Soap Book*, I recommended a 15.5 percent discount; I now use 10 percent. This provides a good approximation of the amount of sodium hydroxide required, but you will still have to experiment.

## Working with a Combination of Oils

The SAP value calculations outlined earlier were for saponifying a single oil. But a soapmaker will never use just a single fat or oil — you will always combine fats and oils to achieve the desired effect. To determine how much base to use in a soap formula that contains several fats and oils, you must calculate the SAP value for the entire mixture of fats and oils. A simple calculation based on combined weight can be made, as follows.

Suppose you wish to combine 5 pounds of olive oil, 3 pounds of coconut oil, and 2 pounds of palm oil. How much sodium hydroxide should you use? Note that the total weight of the oils is 10 pounds, of which 50 percent is olive, 30 percent is coconut, and 20 percent is palm.

Following are the steps to take to figure this amount:

1. Determine the SAP value for the mixture of oils. Using the SAP values chart and the percentage by weight each oil contributes to the whole mixture, calculate the combined SAP value.

   $$.5(189.7) + .3(268) + .2(199.1) = 215$$

2. Multiply the total weight of the oils by the combined SAP value to determine the amount of potassium hydroxide required.

   10 pounds x .215 (215 ÷ 1,000) = 2.15 pounds

3. Multiply 2.15 pounds (the amount of potassium hydroxide required) by the fraction $40/56.1$ to determine the amount of sodium hydroxide required for complete saponification.

   2.15 pounds x $40/56.1$ = 1.53 pounds (of sodium hydroxide)

4. Multiply the result from step 3 by 90 percent (to reflect the 10 percent discount I typically apply to leave some unsaponified fats and oils) to find your final amount of required sodium hydroxide.

   1.53 pounds x 90 percent = 1.38 pounds

Again, remember that this 10 percent discount means that excess fat will be left in your soap, too much of which causes rancidity. If you have this problem, you would notice it after six to twelve months. Fortunately, there is a solution. Adding preservatives — and natural preservatives are available — can postpone rancidity.

I have noticed that the combined SAP values of all of my mixtures are all very close to each other. Indeed, almost all of my SAP values come to within 3 percent of each other.

## SAP VALUES OF COMMON FATS AND OILS

*(When a chart lists a range of SAP values, I always use the average.)*

| Fat or Oil | SAP Value | Fat or Oil | SAP Value |
|---|---|---|---|
| Almond (sweet) oil | 192.5 | Neem oil | 194.5 |
| Apricot kernel oil | 190.0 | Olive oil | 189.7 |
| Avocado oil | 187.5 | Palm kernel oil | 219.9 |
| Babassu oil | 247.0 | Palm oil | 199.1 |
| Beef tallow | 197.0 | Peanut oil | 192.1 |
| Borage oil | 188.0 | Pumpkin seed oil | 193.0 |
| Calendula oil | 190.0 | Rosa mosqueta rosehip seed oil | 193.0 |
| Canola/Rapeseed oil | 174.7 | | |
| Castor oil | 180.3 | Safflower oil | 192.0 |
| Cocoa butter | 193.8 | Sesame oil | 187.9 |
| Coconut oil | 268.0 | Shea butter (African karite butter) | 180.0 |
| Corn oil | 192.0 | | |
| Evening primrose oil | 191.0 | Soybean oil | 190.6 |
| Hazelnut oil | 195.0 | Sunflower seed oil | 188.7 |
| Hemp seed oil | 192.8 | Wheat germ oil | 185.0 |
| Jojoba oil | 97.5 | **Wax** | |
| Kukui nut oil | 190.0 | Beeswax | 88–100 |
| Laurate canola oil | 219.0 | Lanolin (wool fat) | 82–130 |
| Lard | 194.6 | Lecithin | 110–140 |
| Macadamia nut oil | 195.0 | | |

**Note on Castor Oil:** Because of its higher molecular weight, castor oil has a lower SAP value and, in theory, requires less sodium hydroxide for saponification. But castor oil, with its high ricinoleic-acid content, has its own set of rules. Ricinoleic acid has an unusual molecular arrangement, pulling castor oil into some additional bonding within the soap pan. More sodium hydroxide is required to accommodate the extra workload. When a formula calls for over 15 percent castor oil, use a superfatting discount of 5 percent, instead of a 10 percent superfatting discount.

**Note on Waxes:** Beeswax, lanolin, and lecithin are not triglycerides and contain high percentages of unsaponifiables. At best, half of these substances participate in the normal soapmaking reaction. The remainder of material either remains in its original state in the final soap, or it participates in other chemical reactions. Limit the use of these materials in cold-process soapmaking (see pages 193–194).

## EVALUATION OF FATS AND OILS

When you purchase a fat or oil, ask your supplier for a material safety data sheet, commonly referred to as an MSDS. An MSDS lists a product's physical data; fire, explosion, and reactivity hazard data; health hazard information (including hazardous ingredients); precautions for safe handling and use; and waste disposal methods. It is worth learning how to read an MSDS so that you can more reliably anticipate what your soap characteristics will be.

### Iodine Value

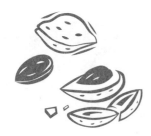

The iodine value measures a fat or oil's saturation. It represents the amount of iodine chloride the fat or oil can absorb, expressed in centigrams of iodine chloride accepted per gram of oil or fat. Saturated fats have low iodine values, and unsaturated oils have high iodine values. Unsaturated oils can absorb more iodine chloride than saturated, which have more of their bonds full. Fats with low iodine values, such as coconut oil, palm oil, palm kernel oil, babassu oil, beef tallow, and lard, usually produce the hardest soaps.

### Peroxide Value

Peroxide value measures the level of chemical change in a material. It is a good indicator of whether an oil is fresh or aged. Oxygen is a most active element, and it reacts easily to form unstable compounds. One kind of peroxide is formed when oxygen attaches itself to the double bonds of unsaturated fatty acids. The resulting carbon chains with peroxides are precursors of rancidity and contribute to spoilage.

The peroxide value of a fat or oil is determined by measuring the amount of iodine that its peroxides are able to liberate from potassium iodide in an acetic-acid solution. Technically, the peroxide value represents the milliequivalents of peroxide (an oxide containing a high percentage of oxygen) per kilogram of sample that oxidizes potassium iodide under specifically defined conditions. Because it measures the

## IODINE VALUES OF COMMON FATS AND OILS

| Fat or Oil | Iodine Value |
|---|---|
| *(amount of iodine chloride, in centigrams, dissolved in 1 gram of oil)* | |
| Almond (sweet) oil | 105.0 |
| Apricot kernel oil | 102.5 |
| Avocado oil | 80.0 |
| Babassu oil | 15.5 |
| Beef tallow | 49.5 |
| Castor oil | 85.5 |
| Coconut oil | 10.4 |
| Jojoba oil | 85.0 |
| Kukui nut oil | 165.0 |
| Lard | 58.6 |
| Macadamia nut oil | 195.0 |
| Olive oil | 81.1 |
| Palm kernel oil | 37.0 |
| Palm oil | 54.2 |
| Peanut oil | 93.4 |
| Soybean oil | 130.0 |
| Wheat germ oil | 125.0 |

content of reactive oxygen in a particular fat or oil, it reflects a fat or oil's propensity toward rancidity. The higher the peroxide value, the more prone to rancidity.

Triglycerides can become rancid over time, as they are exposed to air and react with oxygen to form unstable compounds. A rancid fat or oil has an unpleasant odor.

## Oxidation

When oils or fats are exposed to air, or when soaps superfatted with an excess of neutral oils or fats (triglycerides, diglycerides, or monoglycerides) are exposed to air, oxygen in the air reacts with available atoms to form new, less stable compounds. This is called oxidation. The addition of oxygen at or near the double bonds of the hydrocarbon chains creates peroxides, which are transitory and decompose or react with other compounds to form aldehydes, the compounds responsible for rancid flavor and odor. Low-molecular-weight fatty acids are formed. Rancidity can develop even when no more than .1 percent of the fat or oil undergoes oxidation.

Oxidation often takes place in two distinct phases. During the first stage, oxidation is relatively slow to begin; once it does, however, the reaction moves into the second stage, during which oxidation quickly accelerates. A rancid smell coincides with the beginning of the second phase, and it is not long before brown areas of rancidity nearly cover the bar. It is thought that the more saturated fats and oils are less affected by the early phases of oxidation, but that when it does strike, its progress is accelerated. Unsaturated oils begin to deteriorate quickly, but degrade more slowly over a longer period of time.

The rate of rancidification of fats and oils varies according to a number of factors, all of which contribute to rancidity: the number and position of double bonds within the fatty acids; the presence or absence of antioxidants or prooxidants (the presence of tocopherols, or vitamin E, in lard and tallow offers these fats some protection); fragrance; free fatty acid content; peroxide content; climate (temperature and moisture content); exposure to light; and exposure to ozone. Saturated as well as unsaturated fatty acids are vulnerable to oxidation, though stearic and oleic acids are more stable than linoleic and linolenic acids.

Antioxidants, such as grapefruit seed extract and tocopherols, react with any free oxygen molecules, temporarily tying them up and therefore prolonging the life of a soap.

## Titer

The value known as titer is one indicator of a fat or oil's ability to produce hard soap. It is the temperature at which the mixed fatty acids from a particular fat or oil solidify. A fat or oil with a high titer produces harder bars of soap. Titer reveals more about an oil's soap characteristics than does the melting point of the neutral oil. Technically, titer is the solidification temperature, expressed in degrees Centigrade, of mixed fatty acids. It is determined by cooling down melted fatty acids and noting the highest temperature reached before they solidify. As well as being an indicator of a soap's hardness or softness then, titer helps us to gauge our soapmaking temperatures — according to the points at which fats and oils begin to solidify.

## Acid Value

Free fatty acids (FFA) are those fatty acids within a fat or an oil that are not chemically bound to other fatty acids and glycerol as triglycerides. Most free fatty acids are removed from the oil during refinement, as they contribute to premature rancidity. Alkali refining of fats and oils (also called refinement — ridding the fats and oils of many free fatty acids by reacting them with an alkali to form a soap that is later washed from the oil) reduces the free fatty-acid content to the minimum standard of .05–.15 percent. The acid value is based on the percentage of free fatty acids present in a particular fat or oil; the soapmaker looks for fresh material with a low acid value. Technically, acid value is expressed as the number of milligrams of potassium hydroxide needed to neutralize the fatty acid in 1 gram of fatty material. It is important that this measurment be relatively low, as too high a percentage of free fatty acids accelerates decay.

## Raw Color (Lovibond)

The Lovibond method, as well as other methods, grades the color and clarity of different fats and oils. The degree of color is measured after a sample is heated to 10°C (50°F) above its melting point. It helps you to gauge the color of the final bar by telling you the shades of the fats and oils ahead of time. Fats and oils are best tested for color after refinement, when the comparison of quality is a more reliable indicator. Comparing crude oils is less helpful. The color in better-quality crude oil often comes from natural carotenoids — the pigments responsible for yellow and red colors — that are easily removed during refinement and bleaching. Lower-grade crude oils retain much of their dark color even after refinement, as the degraded materials that produce the dark color are not easily removed. Since dark color is often an indicator of a degraded product, this measure of color also helps you to determine purity.

## Refractive Index

The refractive index is a way to measure a fat or an oil's clarity at a given temperature — often 50°C (122°F). The lower values on the refractive index are assigned to those fats and oils that are optically more clear and less cloudy. Such oils as coconut and babassu have lower values. Higher values are assigned to more turbid fats and oils, such as tung oil, mustard oil, niger seed oil, and perilla oil. At a quick glance the numbers reveal little, for the values all fall between 1.443 and 1.5174. Only by comparison are the numbers helpful to the soapmaker. Usually, as the lengths and the molecular weights of the fatty acid chains of fats and oils increase, the refractive index increases. Some exceptions include coconut oil, babassu oil, and palm kernel oil, which contain high percentages of shorter-chain fatty acids with *high* molecular weights. This unusual composition leaves these three oils with smaller values despite higher molecular weights.

## Unsaponifiables

The materials within a fat or an oil that do not react with alkali to form soap are called unsaponifiables, and are measured as a percentage by weight of the total fats and oils. They are often considered impurities, and some unsaponifiables are removed along with the free fatty acids when the fats and oils are refined. But unlike free fatty acids, a certain percentage of unsaponifiables left in the fats and oils can be beneficial. Some have been known to act as catalysts by decreasing tracing times, and one in particular — the hydrocarbon squalene — possesses antioxidant qualities. Other helpful unsaponifiables include carotenoids, tocopherols, and sterols. (Tocopherols, also known as vitamin E, are antioxidants as well.) Most fats and oils contain between .5 and 2 percent unsaponifiables. Waxes contain much higher percentages: Lanolin has around 40 percent, and beeswax, 50 percent.

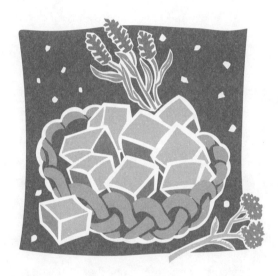

# Soapmaking in the Marketplace

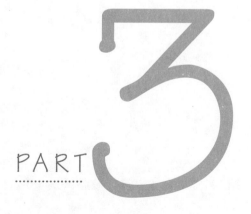

# PART 3

# CHAPTER 14
## Soapmaking Online

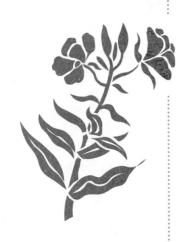

While I was raising children and oblivious to over a decade of technological advances, computer science was reinventing itself annually. Not until just a few years ago had I even heard of a modem.

In the not-so-distant past, for most of us the soapmaking adventure was a solitary one. For me, there was just the kitchen and some books. One experiment after another failed, too often after midnight, though I was always sure that good soap was right around the corner. That next slight adjustment would do the trick. But for a long while, I was wrong. And no one was talking.

Today, people are talking a blue streak. They're warm and sharing and truly eager to talk soap. These are the folks from all over the world who share soapmaking with one another using online providers.

## What Does "Online" Mean?

Computers can be connected to one another and to large central servers through modems. *Modem* stands for "modulator/demodulator"; it is a small device that converts digital computer language into sounds that can travel through phone lines, then back into digital language. Modems enable computers to communicate with one another. A lone computer can store, retrieve, and compute, but it cannot communicate with other computers. A computer with a modem, however, can access other computers with modems. These connected computers share information, search one another's databases, and store any gathered information. Soapmakers can now access a wide range of soapmaking resources.

# WHAT IS THE INTERNET?

Today's Internet evolved out of a 1968 military project called Arpanet, a computer network designed by the United States Department of Defense to allow for the relay of critical information in the event of a nuclear disaster. But after a few years in operation, it became clear that Arpanet alone would not be able to meet the demands. Thus this military project broadened its scope: In an attempt to serve millions of people, many thousands of networks would be connected to form a worldwide Internet. No longer was this system limited to government and university use.

Now, with millions of people who want access to the Internet, a variety of companies and organizations have carved out opportunities to serve these needs profitably. Some provide Internet access only and are known as Internet service providers (often referred to as ISPs). Others have compiled private libraries of information and private lines of communication that they provide, along with Internet access, for their account holders. These companies are known as online information services, or online providers.

## What Does Online Access Offer the Soapmaker?

Internet service providers offer only Internet access. In contrast, online providers, such as Compuserve, America Online, and Prodigy, offer Internet access plus a variety of private resources not found on the Internet. These companies feature special-interest forums that cannot be accessed by anyone other than account holders. Subscribers with an interest in soapmaking can plug into a soapmaking zone to "talk" with one another about soap, browse through a library of stored information, search for related online sites, and read the many messages posted daily. A beginning soapmaker can now "post" any question or observation for others to retrieve and address.

Online providers charge higher fees than do the Internet service providers, but the soapmaker may want more than just Internet access. Both beginning and experienced soapmakers enjoy interaction with other soapmakers. More than just a retrieval system, online communication is an arena in which folks can bounce ideas, questions, frustrations, and successes off one another. No question is ridiculous; it's probably been asked before. All responses are designed to help or to humor, and the spirit of cooperation is ever present.

Soapmaking forums periodically host "soap swaps," the exchange by mail of some favorite bars, often around a theme, such as herbal soaps, baby soaps, or milk soaps. This is an inexpensive, fun way to sample a variety of soaps and to get constructive, good-spirited feedback from others. Behind every screen name and each message posted is a real person. When the soaps arrive, each computer friend becomes three-dimensional.

No longer must beginners read and reread the soapmaking instructions, straining to see what they might have overlooked. Soapmaking online is a way to bear one another's burdens and minimize wheel spinning. The solitary adventure can become a shared journey.

## Mailing Lists

Mailing lists are discussion groups carried out by electronic mail and handled by a computer program that receives and sends messages from one subscriber in the group to all of the others. They are large e-mail loops through which participants can send messages to everyone in the group at once, instead of sending individual messages one at a time.

As interest dictates, a founder assigns a name to a special-interest mailing list and usually oversees the list as an administrator. But the mailing list is actually managed by the computer program that runs it, such as Listserv, Listproc, or Majordomo. It is the program itself that keeps track of the subscribers, receives and sends all messages to all subscribers, and handles requests to add or delete addresses.

Rather than posting a message to just one online provider's soapmaking forum, the soapmaker can send a message that will be read by soapmakers from a variety of online and Internet service providers. The input is more diversified. You can also choose to receive your messages as separate pieces of e-mail or in the form of a digest, a collection of all of that day's messages into one long e-mail. Mailing lists tend to generate a tremendous amount of mail, so beware of overload and read selectively.

## Internet Service Providers

Soapmakers who may not have the time or the budget to subscribe to online providers often choose Internet service providers to receive less expensive Internet access. There are no frills, such as daily news updates, libraries, or forums, but Internet access alone is a world of access, and your online address enables you to participate in mailing lists.

Though there are fewer opportunities for discussion, information concerning any issue imaginable can probably be found through some Internet address. All Internet users have access to web pages, information organized into files and given an Internet address for easy access. Web pages are designed by individuals, businesses, libraries, and universities to make the public aware of their existence. Some pages educate; others sell products. A health organization may set up its own web page to educate the public. A company selling natural soaps may design a web page to advertise.

Some Internet providers also offer access to Usenet groups, also known as newsgroups, collections of discussion groups centered around particular topics, and created as interest and demand dictate within companies and organizations. These groups, unlike web pages on the Internet, can field questions and are codified by topic — business, science, or education, for instance. Soapmakers with Usenet capability (not all Internet service providers offer it) can post questions at Usenet sites, though the response rate is sometimes low. The beauty of the soapmaking forums offered by online providers is the ongoing discussion. Responses are quick and the conversations seem to never end. Usenet groups address inquiries, but they are not designed to be chatty.

The Internet offers the soapmaker a constantly expanding international encyclopedia and marketplace at the touch of a keyboard. You can create on it a web page advertising and selling your soaps; search it for soap-related businesses and organizations, or potential suppliers of raw materials; and use it to research soap-related issues. The opportunities grow daily.

## ONE FINAL THOUGHT

Some opportunities are best utilized when they are less utilized. Online access is available twenty-four hours a day, and like any good thing, it can seduce people into excess. I researched only a small part of this large world, yet within the soapmaking forums alone I saw signs of people devoting valuable chunks of their time to reading and responding to snappy talk. Retrieve and share tips and anecdotes, but beware that gossip and chatter affect online groups just as they affect people offline.

Fortunately, once you get the hang of it, you can quickly skim forum and mailing list posts for the gist of their messages. Rather than spending your time reading each message from start to finish, I advise scanning them for tidbits of information. When I spend time online, I skim the list of posts by subject, ignoring those less relevant and reading only those of interest. Just as an e-mail is less nourishing and satisfying than a good, long handwritten letter, these messages can read like notes being passed in class. Like any other resource, online communication is more helpful and nurturing when it is used discriminatingly.

# CHAPTER 15
## Starting a Soap Business

$S$ince the publication of *The Natural Soap Book,* one of the questions asked of me most often is, "I'm thinking of starting a soap business — do you have any tips?" Well, I do. Starting a business is a legal decision, a business decision, and a personal decision.

Let's focus first on the personal issues. Be very clear why you may want to start a soap business. Making soaps can be fun. Experimentation can be fun. Talking to soapmakers can be fun. But operating a soap business, or any business, is not necessarily fun. It can become a grind. And it can interfere with your other responsibilities as a parent, spouse, wage earner, or human being.

My first piece of advice, then, is to not start a soap business unless you are strongly motivated by the desire to make soap for profit and are prepared to dedicate a very substantial amount of your time and energy to that goal.

My second piece of advice is not to start a soap business unless you are prepared to aggressively market your products. The difference between business failure and success is not likely to depend upon how good a bar you make or even how economically you make it. Rather, success requires aggressive marketing. It means attending weekend craft fairs and trade shows, soliciting store owners, contracting with sales representatives, and advertising. If the private thrill of creating a new scent or the quiet satisfaction of making an aesthetically fine batch of soap is what it's all about for you, then I applaud. But that won't build a successful soap business. If you do not enjoy the process of selling, or are not prepared to concentrate on the process of selling, or are not partnering with someone who will focus on selling, then don't start a soapmaking business.

My third and final piece of personal advice is always to question whether you want to continue the business. There is nothing wrong with starting a business and later deciding to quit. Too often we let ourselves become trapped in a routine that does not suit us. If your business is unprofitable, lack of funds will eventually force you to quit. But even if you are not hemorrhaging cash, do not be slow to do what's best for you. If your parenting is suffering, or you are perpetually tense, or your mood is getting dark, ask yourself whether the economic reward is worth it. If you are embarrassed to quit because you think people will think less of you, don't worry. Nobody really cares.

That's enough preaching. Let's assume that you've decided to start a soapmaking business and want to get a feel for the legal and business issues. There are seven key issues to address:

◆ Whether to operate the business as a sole proprietorship
  or as a corporation
◆ How to form a corporation
◆ How to choose a name
◆ What is meant by income tax planning
◆ When sales taxes must be collected
◆ What insurance coverage is available
◆ Which FDA regulations apply

## CHOICE OF ENTITY

The very first legal question is what sort of entity will technically own and operate the business. You have many different alternatives: A sole proprietorship, a general partnership, a limited partnership, a C corporation, an S corporation, or a limited liability company. Each has its own legal ramifications, so your decision should be deliberate and well informed.

If you simply start making and selling soap without creating any separate entity, then you will be known as a "sole proprietor" and your business will be legally classified as a sole proprietorship. A proprietor is an owner. A sole proprietor is the only owner. If you are a sole proprietor, then you, individually, own the raw materials you purchase, the equipment you use, and the soaps you sell. If you have employees, you are their employer.

You do not have to operate your business as a sole proprietorship, however. You can choose to form a legal entity that owns and operates the business. You, in turn, own the entity. For example, if you form a corporation, the corporation owns and operates the soapmaking business; you own the corporation and are called a stockholder or shareholder. There are four different kinds of entities from which to choose:

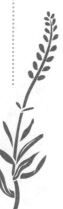

- ◆ General partnership
- ◆ Limited partnership
- ◆ Corporation
- ◆ Limited liability company

There are occasions when a general partnership, limited partnership, or limited liability company makes sense, especially if there will be more than one owner of the business. But for most, the likely choice will be either a sole proprietorship or a corporation.

The biggest advantage of a corporation is that it limits the liability of you, the owner. Theoretically, if your corporation runs out of money and cannot afford to pay its bills, its creditors — mostly suppliers — will simply never get paid. Unless you, the shareholder, personally guarantee a corporate debt, you never have to pay it off personally. Similarly, if an employee of your corporation negligently mixes a batch of soap and creates a bar with too much lye and a customer sues your corporation, your corporation may lose, but you will not be forced to use your personal assets to cover any settlement or judgment. Limiting liability is the most common reason for forming a corporation.

This advantage is somewhat less applicable to a beginning soapmaker. Suppliers are likely to sell to you COD or require you to personally guarantee your corporation's debts. And if your corporation has no other employees, then any negligent manufacturing will be attributable to you personally as well as to your corporation. Thus, both you and the corporation will be sued, and both will be liable.

Accordingly, creating a corporation is not likely to be highly advantageous until you have employees. And there are some disadvantages to consider. For example, forming a corporation will probably cost you around $500 up front. Then every year your corporation will need to file certain documents with the state. It will have to prepare corporate tax returns — a federal tax return, a state tax return, and, depending upon where you live, a local tax return. Between the extra legal fees, the accounting fees, and just plain aggravation, forming a corporation probably does not make good sense — again, until you grow and hire employees.

## FORMING A CORPORATION

If you choose to form a corporation, it is easy to do. Pretty much all it takes is to file a single document called a charter (or, in some states, the articles of incorporation) with the secretary of state of the state in which you live, along with a filing fee. The charter is usually a very short document — often only one page. It is required to contain certain information and usually does not contain more than the required minimum. The state filing fee is apt to be in the $100 range. If you engage a lawyer, the legal fee for preparing the charter and other organizational documents is likely to be in the $500 range.

### Establishing The Basics

Filing a charter with the state creates a corporation — but only a shell. The corporation does not yet have any shareholders, or a board of directors, or any officers, or even any assets. That's why the next step is for you to contribute money and/or property to the corporation in exchange for stock. This requires subscribing for stock, preparing a bill of sale transferring ownership of the contributed property from you to the corporation, and preparing a stock certificate.

You are now the sole shareholder of your corporation. As sole shareholder, you'll elect a board of directors. Most likely, you'll be the sole director. The board of directors (you) then elects the officers. Most

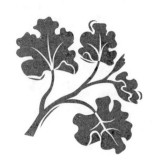

states — maybe all states — require that there be at least a president and a secretary, and the same person cannot be both. You'll probably elect yourself president and choose a friend or spouse as secretary.

Your corporation will need to apply for a taxpayer identification number. Whereas people have social security numbers, corporations and other entities have taxpayer identification numbers. You need to apply to the IRS for this number by filling out Treasury Form SS-4. You can also apply for the number over the phone by giving the same information that is requested on the form.

Your corporation should also adopt a set of bylaws. This is a relatively long document explaining how the shareholders meet and vote, how the directors are chosen, meet, and vote, and what the officers' duties are. Every business lawyer has a set of standard bylaws on a word processor. The bylaws are not filed with the state; it's a private document.

Finally, your corporation will need to open a bank account. It will get a corporate checkbook. You'll probably want only one signatory on the checks — you.

Again, all of this legal work will probably cost you around $500. Most of the paperwork is on a word processor, so not much of your lawyer's time will be required. The fee generally covers the time your lawyer spends getting information from you and explaining to you how corporations work.

## Choosing a Name

If you form a corporation, the corporate charter will state the name you've chosen for it. So long as this name does not too closely resemble another name on file with the secretary of state, you will be permitted to use it. If you choose a name identical to another corporation's, or so close that it is likely to cause confusion, the secretary of state will not file your charter. You should call the secretary of state's office (located in your state's capital) before you mail the charter and ask if your desired name is available.

Even if you operate as a sole proprietorship and not as a corporation, you can operate under another name. This is known as a trade name.

Corporations can have trade names too. You've heard of d/b/a's. That stands for "doing business as," which prefaces a trade name.

You may not have to file any special document with the state if you want to use a trade name. But if you want to protect your exclusive rights to use the trade name and keep others from using it, you'd be wise to register it with the secretary of state. This requires a nominal fee — probably in the $20 range.

If you want to establish exclusive rights to use the name across the entire country, you'll need to federally register it. This is a somewhat bigger to-do and may require the services of a copyright attorney.

## Income Tax Planning

This topic is so huge and so technical that you'll positively have to rely upon a tax attorney or tax accountant for advice. Still, there are some basics worth understanding.

If you form a corporation, you'll need to choose between being a C corporation and being an S corporation. The letters refer to the subchapter of the Internal Revenue Code under which a corporation is taxed. A C corporation pays its own taxes and is subject to corporate tax rates. An S corporation does not pay income tax. Instead, its taxable income flows through to the shareholders (you) and is includable on your individual tax return.

You are likely to be better off in the short run and the long run as an S corporation. Your corporation must file an election to be an S corporation, and the shareholders (you) must sign their consent. This is all done on Treasury Form 2553, which must be filed within two and a half months after the beginning of the corporation's tax year to be effective for the current tax year.

In general, being a sole proprietorship offers a tax advantage over being a C corporation. When you file your tax return as a sole proprietorship, your profit and loss are reported on Schedule C of Form 1040. Being an S corporation comes much closer to being taxable as a sole proprietorship.

When you first start your soap business, you're likely to have losses. From a tax standpoint, losses are good if you can deduct them from taxable income. If you are a sole proprietor, for example, and you and your spouse are otherwise in a 36 percent tax bracket, a $10,000 loss will reduce your joint taxable income by $10,000 and save you $3,600 in taxes (36 percent of $10,000). The same holds true if your corporation is an S corporation and loses $10,000. However, if your corporation is a C corporation, you cannot deduct its loss on your tax return; it can only be deducted in later years when (and if) it ever earns a taxable profit.

One particularly important warning for business soapmakers is to avoid being treated by the Internal Revenue Service, for tax purposes, as a hobbyist. If your activity is treated as only a hobby, then you will be entitled to deduct expenses only up to the amount of your revenue. For example, if you receive revenue of $5,000 but spend $7,000, you'll only be able to deduct $5,000 of those expenses. The result is zero income. But if you are a business, you'll be able to deduct the full $7,000, resulting in a net loss of $2,000. If you are in a 36 percent tax bracket, the net loss will actually save $720 in taxes (36 percent of $2,000).

To avoid being treated as a hobbyist, run your business like a business. Keep detailed accounting records. Be able to demonstrate how hard you are working and how diligently you are focused on earning a profit. No IRS agent who tried manning a trade show booth for a three-day weekend could believe you were making soap for fun! Even if you never earn a profit, it is possible to be treated for tax purposes as a business. The Internal Revenue Code presumes that if you were profitable in at least three of your last five years, you are in business. But this presumption is rebuttable, and more important, failing the test does not mean you are a hobbyist.

## Paying Sales Taxes

Most, if not all, states impose a tax on retail sales. The tax is to be paid by the retail customer and collected by the vendor. If you collect sales tax, you'll need to fill out a state sales tax return — probably every three months — and pay the state what you collected (or should have collected). Even if a vendor does not collect the tax from its customers, it may still owe the tax to the state department of revenue.

The tax is imposed only on retail sales. In general, there is no tax on wholesale sales, casual sales, or interstate sales.

When you sell soaps to a retail store, to a distributor, or to any other entity that will simply resell the soap, you will not need to collect sales tax. Only the final sale in the chain — to the retail customer — is subject to sales tax.

It is possible to sell soaps to the end user without incurring a sales tax, however. This exception is for so-called "casual sales." If you sell your lawn mower to a neighbor, there is no sales tax. You are not in the business of selling lawn mowers and such sales are infrequent. Similarly, if you are not in the soapmaking business, but occasionally sell a few bars to friends, you can legitimately rely upon the casual sale exception and not charge sales tax. (But note that when you sell a car, even though the sale is casual it is still likely to be subject to sales tax; that's because there is typically an exception to the exception for casual sales of motor vehicles.)

Finally, interstate mail-order sales are not subject to state sales tax. This tax break is attributable to the U.S. Constitution, which prohibits states from interfering with interstate commerce.

# CHAPTER 16
## Insuring Your Business

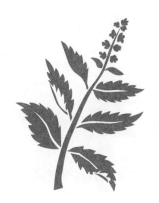

There are three risks you want to be insured against:

**1.** What if you damage your house while making soap? (I consider this risk extraordinarily remote, except while making transparent soap, at which time the risk is simply remote.)
**2.** What if your soap injures someone who uses it?
**3.** Who pays your legal fees if someone sues you?

The answer, under your homeowner's policy, is likely to depend upon whether you are in the business of soapmaking. My own policy clearly states that there is no coverage for "personal injury, bodily injury or property damage arising out of business pursuits." The term *business* is defined to include "any activity aimed at providing a product or service with the anticipation of a profit from the enterprise."

A straightforward, literal reading of this tells me the following: If I am just a hobbyist, even if I occasionally sell some soap, I am probably covered by my homeowner's policy; if I am in the business of trying to make a profit from soapmaking, I am probably not covered by my homeowner's policy. In the latter case, I would need to purchase separate insurance coverage for my business. I am advised by insurance agents that there are no riders to homeowner policies that cover the additional risks of operating a business.

## WHAT TO LOOK FOR IN A POLICY

Be very wary of inexpensive insurance policies that are marketed as specialty policies for crafters or in-home businesses. Their applications are seductively simple and their premiums are comfortably low. There is a reason for this.

Before you buy a policy, make sure that you understand what coverage you are getting. Specialty policies may not adequately protect you from the three risks listed on the preceding page. For example, you should have product liability coverage (protecting you from liability for injuries caused by your soap product). Some specialty policies, however, only cover liability for injuries to people who slip and fall on your premises. Such coverage is important when you operate a retail business and have many customers walking through your premises. But it is not so important if you are manufacturing soap alone in your home.

Even with respect to coverage for property damage, specialty policies are likely to fall far short of what the soapmaker needs. Such policies routinely cover damage to certain personal property — such as equipment. But they may not cover damage to your real property (the house). Thus, if you damage your house while making transparent soap for your business, you may not be covered for most of the loss. Possibly, only damage to soapmaking equipment in the room where you make your soap will be covered. This means your scales, your spatulas, and maybe your computer.

Also, make sure that the insurance company has a duty to defend you if you are sued for a covered liability. Even if the claim against you is weak or frivolous, legal fees can run into the tens of thousands of dollars.

My final caveat with respect to specialty policies is to read the application aggressively. Pretend that you are the lawyer for the insurance company and are trying to find an excuse to not honor your insurance claim after a problem arises. If any of your answers on the application are inaccurate, coverage will be denied. These specialty insurers will not investigate your answers on the front end. (That's one reason their premiums are so low — because their underwriting costs are so low.) Rather, they'll investigate only when you most need them — when you are trying to collect on a claim. Note that I have not yet read an application for specialty coverage that did not include at least one question or condition that disqualified me from coverage.

If you want insurance coverage, and if your homeowner's policy does not cover you, and if you agree that the specialty coverage is inadequate, then you will need to purchase a conventional commercial and general liability policy. This will be expensive.

# CHAPTER 17
## Federal Regulation of Soapmaking

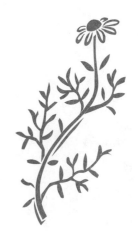

For purposes of avoiding federal regulation, you want to be a soap-maker, not a cosmetic maker, and certainly not a drug maker. Surprisingly, many of today's small soapmakers are not considered soapmakers under federal law and are therefore subject to certain federal regulations. Less surprising is that most are not aware of this.

The federal law begins with two statutes: the Food, Drug & Cosmetic Act, adopted by Congress in 1938, and the Fair Packaging & Labeling Act, adopted by Congress in 1939. These statutes are then administered by the Food and Drug Administration (FDA), which adopts regulations. These regulations have the force of law even though they were not adopted by Congress. Most of the details discussed in this chapter come from the FDA regulations, not the original statutes.

## AVOIDING REGULATIONS

There are two ways to avoid these federal rules. The first way is to simply not manufacture soaps for sale or distribution. If you make soap simply for yourself and your family, just as a hobby, these rules do not apply.

The second way to avoid the federal rules is to manufacture what the law considers a soap. The law applies to "cosmetics," which are statutorily defined to include "articles intended to be rubbed . . . or otherwise applied to the human body . . . for cleaning . . . except that such term shall not include soap." The statute does not define "soap," but the FDA regulations do. To qualify as a soap, and therefore be exempt from federal cosmetic regulations, your soap must satisfy *both* of the following conditions:

**1.** The detergent properties of the soap must be due exclusively to the alkali–fatty acid compounds in the soap. This requirement is easily met. In fact, I do not know of any cold-process soap that does not satisfy it. All of the soap recipes in this book and in *The Natural Soap Book* clearly meet this requirement.

**2.** The soap must be labeled, sold, and represented only as soap. This is the big one – the requirement many soapmakers unwittingly violate. If you claim any medicinal or curative powers, your soap ceases to be soap under the law. If you claim that your soap moisturizes, your soap is no longer a soap. If you claim that your soap helps people with eczema, your soap is not a soap.

## MEETING REGULATIONS FOR COSMETICS

If federal law appertaining to cosmetics applies to your soapmaking, you will need to concern yourself with several rules, the most important ones being the following:

**Labeling.** If federal law classifies your soap as a cosmetic, you will need to label it. The label must indicate several things. First is the net weight of the contents in ounces. The net weight may also be expressed using metric units (i.e., grams), but even in this case, ounces must be disclosed. The label must also state the name and address of the manufacturer, including the street address, city, state, and zip code. If it is listed in a current telephone directory, though, the street address may be omitted.

Most important, your ingredients must be listed in the order of their predominance. (Color additives and ingredients present at under 1 percent may be listed without regard for predominance. Some ingredients are exempt from disclosure regulations and may be referred to simply as "and other ingredients.") The actual percentages of each ingredient do not have to be included. Also, the ingredients must be identified by the names established or adopted by regulation. The declaration of ingredients must be conspicuously placed on the label so that it is likely to be read by a purchaser; the letters must be at least 1/16 inch (1.5 mm) in height (1/32 inch [0.78 mm] if the total package surface available to bear labeling is less than 12 square inches [77.4 square cm]).

Some soapmakers are under the erroneous impression that a chemical is not an ingredient if it reacted with other chemicals and is thus no longer present in the final product. These soapmakers, for example, do not think that sodium hydroxide need be listed, since there is no sodium hydroxide left in their final bars. They are wrong. *Ingredient* is not defined as a component of the final bar, but as a component used in the manufacturing process. The FDA regulations define the term as "any single chemical entity or mixture used as a component in the manufacture of a cosmetic product." And *manufacture* means "the making of any cosmetic product by chemical, physical, biological, or other procedures." Combining these two definitions clarifies that an ingredient is any single chemical entity or mixture used as a component in the making of any cosmetic product — including sodium hydroxide. The definition clearly anticipates that the manufacturing process may be a chemical one in which an ingredient reacts and is no longer present in the final product.

If the safety of your materials has not been substantiated — for example, if you use a color additive that has not been expressly approved by the FDA — your label may have to include a conspicuous warning: "Warning — the safety of this product has not been determined."

**Color Additives.**  If federal law classifies your soap as a cosmetic, then your color additives must be tested for safety and approved by the FDA. If you use a color additive that has not been approved, your soap will be considered adulterated and in violation of the law. Many of the natural colorants described in chapter 4, such as alkanet root, rose hips, and brazilwood, have not been expressly approved by the FDA.

**Sanitary Production Process.**  If federal law classifies your soap as a cosmetic, then you must manufacture and store it under sanitary conditions and avoid contamination with filth. This is a standard of cleanliness that kitchen soapmakers are not likely to meet. Sanitized equipment, gloves, hairnets, confirmation of weights and measures by a second person, sampling, water testing, absence of tobacco products — these are just a few of the so-called Good Manufacturing Practice Guidelines cosmetic manufacturers are measured against.

**False Claims.**  If federal law classifies your soap as a cosmetic, then you must be especially careful not to make any claims about it that are exaggerated, misleading, or untrue.

# APPENDIX

## Buyer Guides

The first two guides listed below are better suited to the small-scale soap-maker; the third is a much more costly catalog, relating more to large-scale food manufacture, though it is a helpful cross-reference for equipment (borrowing from food industry) and food-grade fats, oils, and nutrients.

**International Buyers Guide**
The Cosmetic, Toiletry, and
    Fragrance Association
1101 17th Street NW Suite 300
Washington, DC 20036-4702
202-331-1770

**DCI Directory Issue**
Drug and Cosmetic Industry
1 East First Street
Duluth, MN 55802

**Food Engineering Master Catalog**
1 Chilton Way
Radnor, PA 19089
610-964-4000

## Suppliers

Water-Soluble Annatto Powder/
Oil-Soluble Annatto Extract
**Freeman Industries, Inc.**
100 Marbledale Road
Tuckahoe, NY 10707
800-666-6454; 914-961-2100

Bee Propolis
**Glorybee Foods**
120 North Seneca
Eugene, Oregon 97402
800-456-7923

Beeswax
**Endless Mountain Apiaries**
RR #2, Box 171-A
New Milford, PA 18834
717-465-3232

Borax (Sodium borate N.F.
powdered, cosmetic grade)
**Spectrum Chemical Manufacturing
    Corporation**
14422 South San Pedro Street
Gardena, CA 90248
800-772-8786

Chlorophyll
**Freeman Industries, Inc.**
100 Marbledale Road
Tuckahoe, NY 10707
800-666-6454; 914-961-2100

Cocoa Butter
**J. W. Hanson Co., Inc.**
144 Woodbury Road
Woodbury, NY 11797
800-767-0477

Colorants
**Alliance Import Co.**
1021 "R" Street
Sacramento, CA 95814
916-920-8658
*(One of the few suppliers of madder root; also alkanet root, annatto seed, and brazilwood.)*

**Herb Products**
11012 Magnolia Boulevard
P.O. Box 898
North Hollywood, CA 91601
818-984-3141

**San Francisco Herb & Natural
    Food Company**
47444 Kato Road
Fremont, CA 94538
800-227-2830

**Wildweeds**
P.O. Box 88
Ferndale, CA 95536
800-553-WILD

Pure Essential Oils/Fragrance Oils
**Aroma Creations, Inc.**
P.O. Box 75506
Seattle, WA 98125
206-363-1608

**Frontier Cooperative Herbs**
3021 78th Street
P.O. Box 299
Norway, IA 52318
800-669-3275

**Lebermuth Company**
P.O. Box 4103
South Bend, IN 46634
800-648-1123

**Sweet Cakes Soaps & Sundries**
39 Brookdale Road
Bloomfield, NJ 07003
973-338-9830

Fats and Oils
**Arista Industries, Inc.**
1082 Post Road
Darien, CT 06820
800-637-6243; Fax: 203-656-0328

**Columbus Foods Company**
800 North Albany
Chicago, IL 60622
800-322-6457

**Fuji Vegetable Oils**
1 Barker Avenue
White Plains, NY 10601
914-761-7900

**Liberty Natural Products, Inc.**
8120 Southeast Stark
Portland, OR 97215
800-289-8427; 503-256-1227

**Living Seed Products**
P.O. Box 10602
Eugene, OR 97440
888-SEED-OIL
(hemp seed oil — from viable seed, hazelnut oil)

**The Ohio Hempery**
7002 State Route 329
Guysville, OH 45735
800-BUY-HEMP
(hemp seed oil — from sterilized seed)

**Oils of Aloha**
66935 Kaukonahua Road
Waialua, HI 96791
800-367-6010
(kukui nut oil, macadamia nut oil)

**Welch, Holme & Clarke Co., Inc.**
7 Avenue L
Newark, NJ 07105
201-465-1200

*Grapefruit Seed Extract*
**Chemie Research**
P.O. Box 181279
Casselberry, FL 32718-1279
407-831-4519

*Ochers*
**New Riverside Ochre Company**
75 Old River Road, Southeast
P.O. Box 460
Cartersville, GA 30120
800-248-0176

*Resins*
**Aroma Creations, Inc.**
P.O. Box 75506
Seattle, WA 98125
206-363-1608

**The Fanning Corporation**
2450 West Hubbard Street
Chicago, IL 60612
800-FANNING
(copaiba balsam)

**Robertet, Inc.**
125 Bauer Drive
P.O. Box 660
Oakland, NJ 07436-3190
201-337-7100

*Scales*
**Chem Lab Supplies**
1060 Ortega Way, Unit C
Placentia, CA 92670
714-630-7902

*Soapmaking Kits*
**Pretty Baby Herbal Soap Co.**
P.O. Box 555
China Grove, NC 28023
800-673-8167

**Summers Past**
15602 Old Highway 80
Flinn Springs, CA 92021
800-390-9969

*Sodium Hydroxide/Potassium Hydroxide*
**American Research Products Company (AMRESCO)**
30175 Solon Industrial Parkway
Solon, OH 44139-4300
800-829-2802; 216-349-1199

**Chem Lab Supplies**
1060 Ortega Way, Unit C
Placentia, CA 92670
714-630-7902

*Transparent Soapmaking Book*
**Catherine Failor**
c/o Rose City Press
4326 S.E. Woodstock Blvd., Suite 374
Portland, OR 97206
503-771-3234

*Vegetable Glycerin*
**Frontier Cooperative Herbs**
3021 78th Street
P.O. Box 299
Norway, IA 52318
800-669-3275

*Vegetable Stearic Acid*
**Henkel Corporation**
Chemicals Group
5051 Estecreek Drive
Cincinnati, OH 45232-1447
800-543-7370
(large quantities only; inquire about local distributors for small purchases)

*Ultramarines*
**Whittaker, Clark & Daniels, Inc.**
1000 Coolidge Street
South Plainfield, NJ 07080
800-732-0562

# INDEX

Page references in *italic* indicate illustrations.
**Bold** page numbers indicate chart/table references.

# RELATED STOREY PUBLISHING TITLES

**The Natural Soapmaking Kit,** from Storey Communications. Packaged in a reusable wooden mold, this kit contains *The Natural Soap Book* and ingredients to make fifteen 3-ounce bars of natural, vegetable-based soaps. Order #0-88266-995-8.

**The Natural Soap Book: Making Herbal and Vegetable-Based Soaps,** by Susan Miller Cavitch. Explores the goodness of soap, homemade without chemical additives and synthetic ingredients. Contains basic recipes as well as ideas on scenting, coloring, cutting, trimming, and wrapping soaps. 192 pages. Paperback. Order #0-88266-888-9.

**The Herbal Body Book: A Natural Approach to Healthier Hair, Skin, and Nails,** by Stephanie Tourles. How to transform common herbs, fruits, and grains into safe, economical, and natural personal care items. Contains more than 100 recipes. 128 pages. Paperback. Order #0-88266-880-3.

**The Essential Oils Book: Creating Personal Blends for Mind & Body,** by Colleen K. Dodt. A rich resource on the many uses of aromatherapy and its applications in everyday life. Spells out simple recipes that anyone can make from ingredients available at a grocery or health food store. 160 pages. Paperback. Order #0-88266-913-3.

**Natural BabyCare: Pure and Soothing Recipes and Techniques for Mothers and Babies,** by Colleen K. Dodt. Offers easy-to-follow instructions for parents to make natural lotions, bath and massage oils, creams, powders, and shampoos that will ensure glowing health and enhance the bond between parent and child. 160 pages. Paperback. Order #0-88266-953-2.

**Milk-Based Soaps: Making Natural, Skin-Nourishing Soap,** by Casey Makela. Extensive coverage of the processes of making milk-based soaps, long recognized for their gentleness and beautifying effects. Step-by-step instructions and distinctive recipes are sure to appeal to soapmakers of all abilities. 96 pages. Paperback. Order #0-88266-984-2.

**Perfumes, Splashes & Colognes: Discovering and Crafting Your Personal Fragrances,** by Nancy M. Booth. Complete instructions for making, packaging, storing, and using specialty perfume fragrances. 160 pages. Paperback. Order #0-88266-985-0.

**The Candlemaker's Companion,** by Betty Oppenheimer. Guides readers step-by-step through both the how and why of candlemaking in the most complete guide ever. 176 pages. Paperback. Order #0-88266-994-X.

**Growing Your Herb Business,** by Bertha Reppert. Practical advice on budgets, locations, business plans, bookkeeping, staffing, inventory, and pricing. 192 pages. Paperback. Order #0-88266-612-6.

These books and other Storey books are available at your bookstore, farm store, garden center, or directly from Storey Publishing, Schoolhouse Road, Pownal, Vermont 05261, or by calling 800-441-5700. Visit our website at www.storey.com.